THE
INSPIRED
YOGA TEACHER

THE ESSENTIAL GUIDE TO
CREATING TRANSFORMATIONAL CLASSES
YOUR STUDENTS WILL LOVE

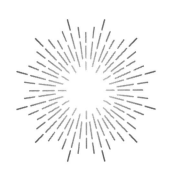

GABRIELLE HARRIS

Thank you for purchasing this book.
Please feel free to use the contents of this book for classes and inspiration.
If you want to reproduce or use material from this book
for teacher trainings, please respect copyright and ask
permission for use. In doing so you are supporting me to
continue writing creative material for teachers' use.
Contact Gabrielle: www.gabrielleharrisyoga.com

This book and the poses within it are not intended as a substitute for
medical advice. Any suggestions are intended to fuel creativity within you
and should be adapted to suit your students. For all matters regarding
health, please seek professional advice. The information given here is
correct to my best knowledge. The author shall not be held responsible
for any loss or damage allegedly arising from the use of this book.

© 2021 Cover design by Susana Cardona
© 2021 Cover picture by Lory Yau
© 2021 Illustrations by Voloshina Svetlana

Note: For economy of words, usually only one side of a sequence is given
and the repetitions or time in the pose is not often stated. I advise testing
the sequences in your own body before trying them in your class.
The sequences or pose sets are not intended as
complete classes but to draw inspiration from.

My Trimurti
The beginning—illustrations by Sveltlana Voloshina, creativemarket.com
The middle—editing by Lindsay Hobbs, topazediting.com
and Meredith Tennant, meredithtennanteditorial.com
The end—book interior and cover design by
Susana Cardona, susanacardona.es

The stunning image of the mala is supplied courtesy of
The Genuine Bead Shop, on Etsy.

Acknowledgements

*I gratefully acknowledge the permissions of the following people
to reprint their work in these pages:*

Deva Premal and Miten, 'Om Asatoma,'
https://devapremalmiten.com/temple/lyrics-chords/

Dr. Scott Lyons' 'Zoom Out' method

Krishna Das, 'Baba Hanuman,'
https://www.krishnadas.com/lyrics/baba-hanuman/

*Schucman, Helen, and William Thetford.
A Course in Miracles. Foundation for Inner Peace, 2007.*

*Ty Burhoe, Invocation, featuring Krishna Das,
Manorama, John Friend, and Amy Ippoliti, Tala Records, 2007.*

*This book is dedicated to my students. Thank you for showing up
and letting me be me. Without you there would be no this.*

Much love, Gabrielle.

TABLE OF

Contents

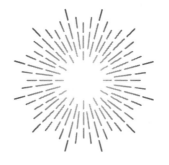

CHAPTER 1

FOR THE TEACHER
17

CHAPTER 2

THE ART OF THEMING
35

CHAPTER 5

STARTING SHAPES

CHAPTER 6

MEANINGFUL MIDDLES

155

*May we appreciate and recognise the lives of
our ancestors whose lives our life was built on.*

*To all of those who have walked
the path before us to pave the way.*

*To our teachers who have lit a candle to guide,
who picked us up when we fell to our knees,
who supported us when we were lost,
who saw within us our beauty and gifts
and believed in us when we had forgotten.*

We give our thanks.

*To the people, to the ancestry to the lineage,
to the land, to all beings, we acknowledge your gifts,
the sacrifices and journeys you made
to support and lead us to this moment.*

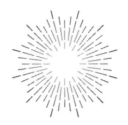

INTRODUCTION

Open your mouth only if what you are about to say is more beautiful than silence.

ARABIC PROVERB

It has been said that the second-greatest fear—after death—is public speaking. To stand up in front of a group of people, share your ideas, teach, guide, inform, and inspire is the everyday job of a teacher. As yoga teachers, we are cheerleaders for our art; choreographers; DJs; body, mind, and spirit caretakers; coaches; 'experts' in our field; equipment waiters; timekeepers; and magicians. All this while finding the words to move and shape people.

It's a complicated job.

And one of the most fulfilling and vital privileges.

Like a sutra or thread, the words we weave form the basis for our class. We need language to communicate our art and science, to inspire others, and to get through the time with a modicum of grace. We need those words on the days when we are tongue-tied, heartbroken, elated, speechless, bewildered, or plain lost. We need them when the sun shines and rainbows surround us and we need them when dark sunglasses barely cover our stained and blurry eyes.

We are the guide for others' breakthroughs and the stakeholders in another's transformation. We are avatars for personal development, authenticity and growth. We are the people holding the advertising billboards for yoga and the keys to unlocking the doors of the heart. We are the conduit for this ancient practice called yoga. And we do all this through the power of words expressed through themes.

You get to set the feeling and tone with your words. Just as you would prepare a table for dinner guests, arrival on the mat is set with what you braid into the opening sequence. Our phrases are bullets and love letters and comfort to those who need them. If you have a few beautiful words, you will turn a worthy experience into an extraordinary one, and this is where transformation happens.

And your students will hear what you have to say precisely when they need to.

You don't need to be a poet, a wordsmith, or an eloquent public speaker to effect change in others; you need to care, you need to ache for change and have dreams, and you need to be you.

This book prompts you to take a fresh look at the shapes we make with our bodies. It reminds us that the little square of rubber under our body is our world, our sanctuary, our life, and all the relationships we have ever had. It is our role model, our teacher, and the container for our thoughts and actions playing out right now.

YOUR SANCTUARY

Lay down your mat.

This is your sanctuary.

It is the white silk flag you raise to yourself when you want to give up or drop out.

It recognises you and will hold your body.

It knows you showed up to be with yourself, to be present, and it permits you to be you. It doesn't mind that you ushered peace out the door or that you are fear-stained. It doesn't see the extra pounds you carried here, your pettiness or regrets.

It will smell like kindness and show you the consequence of truly loving yourself.

So,

take a moment to thank yourself.

This act is another courageous vote of dedication.

It will turn the willpower you never knew you had into an act of fidelity.

Each day you show up to marry your commitment with your faith, you will be rewarded with another footprint in the right direction.

And now that you are ready, this love story begins.

Sutra 1.1

Now Yoga Begins

The practice starts now you are ready.

It starts with meeting all parts of yourself with sweetness and love.

*Wherever you are in your life, whatever you have brought with you to the mat,
this is the perfect place to become curious about the field of yoga which is alive in you now.*

So take your seat, get comfortable, be in your body in present, loving awareness.

And listen to yoga as it is happening now— in your breath, in this posture.

*It is happening in the ordinary way you clean your teeth and brush your hair
and it shines in the extraordinary, a birth, a miracle, the sprouting of a seed.*

Yoga is in the queues, in the cars, in the arguments and in death.

It is in the silences and pauses.

It is found in this moment and in all of your moments.

Yoga is here, and you are yoga.

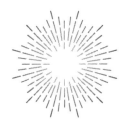

CHAPTER ONE

FOR THE TEACHER

THE SEAT OF THE TEACHER

What we learn and hold within us, our wisdom and knowledge, lie sleeping like genies in a bottle until we bring them to life and display them to the world. When we teach, we animate and awaken the philosophy in the hearts and minds of our students.

The students who consistently show up for our classes are the ones who feel an attraction to the messages we hold, and want to live by these messages. The depths to which we can take another soul will correlate with how intimate we have become with ourself. Once we stop excavating our persona and digging into our psyche, once we stop learning about our *stuff*, the yoga teachings will return to dormancy.

The students who search for meaning in their life will only be able to go as far as you are willing to go, and they will keep attending for as long as you are eager to be a detective of your own life.

Pedagogy is the science behind teaching. It is the study of how we learn best and what conditions facilitate learning.

After more than thirty years as a TESOL (Teaching English to Speakers of Other Languages) and yoga teacher, I have narrowed down the following salient points on teaching and learning.

In some ways, we are all teachers. We live out our lives, and people look to us for example. I don't believe it matters what you do but how you do it. I no longer think you need to know more than anyone else in order to be a good teacher, but you do need to love what you do.

These points are also a guide to living your yoga off the mat.

When I let go of what I am, I become what I might be

LAO TZU

AUTHENTICITY

When we first start teaching, it's easy to imitate a teacher we admire. We arrive in the classroom in the Trojan horse of others' voices, stories, and cues. Sometimes we need to do this to find our feet. Eventually, though, we need to let go of the chameleon in us and respect our individuality. There are as many ways to teach as there are people, so there is no need to silence who we are or force ourselves into the shapes or expectations of others.

In her book, *The Top Five Regrets of the Dying*[1], Bronnie Ware states that the number one regret is 'I wish I'd had the courage to live a life true to myself, not the life others expected of me.'

CONSIDER SATYA

Satya, or being true, is the basis for authentic teaching. The shortcomings, messes, and crevices in our life that we need to wake up to, what we know and don't know, is where satya is buried.

When we honestly look at all our parts, including our strengths, and disentangle ourselves from self-judgement, we become more comfortable with who we are and what we can offer.

If we can't be honest with ourselves first, then we can't be honest in any other part of our life, including what we teach.

Instead of putting a representation of yourself into the world, consider investing more fully in your uniqueness.

TEACH WHAT YOU KNOW

Start where you are with what you have.

The yoga body of information is so vast, it's not possible to understand it all in depth. Working knowledge of the basic principles of all the disciplines can be helpful, such as yoga asana, yoga anatomy, yoga philosophy, Ayurveda, Traditional Chinese Medicine (TCM), and yoga as therapy. Still, it would take many lifetimes to know each of these subjects in

---

[1] Bronnie Ware, *The Top Five Regrets of the Dying: A Life Transformed by the Dearly Departing* (Hay House Inc., 2012).

detail. We may not be doctors, physical therapists, alternative medicine practitioners, or psychologists, but we are teachers, and we can teach what *we* know.

Aim to have a primary connection to or understanding of what you impart rather than a secondary one. A secondary connection is when you have heard or read the information, but you haven't embodied, practised, or fully understood it yet. For example, reading about how to play the piano and playing the piano are two different levels of understanding.

However, at times we may need to attempt teaching something we can't fully do ourselves because, through teaching, we learn ourselves. Remaining one breath, one step, ahead of what the students may know is enough to carry our shortfalls in knowledge. Be aware if this is your intent.

UNDERSTAND THAT THE MORE YOU KNOW, THE LESS YOU KNOW

The paradox of learning is that once we unleash the doors to an enquiry, it is like a hall of mirrors in that it keeps reflecting in all directions. Be okay with your uncertainties, with saying 'I don't know,' and the word 'maybe'. Be okay with unlearning what you have learnt as your knowledge and skills grow and develop.

Here are the stages of learning first developed by Martin M Broadwell in 1969.

+ Unconscious incompetence: the learner is unaware of what they don't know.

+ Conscious incompetence: the learner knows they have a deficit in their knowledge or skills. It is at this stage that learning can start, and mistakes are part of that learning. It is also the stage at which they are most likely to quit.

+ Conscious competence: the learner knows they have the skill but requires concentration to perform the task.

+ Unconscious competence: the learner has enough skills to perform the task with ease as if they are in the flow.

BE ENTHUSIASTIC AND CURIOUS ABOUT YOUR SUBJECT

You don't necessarily need to be an expert in your subject, but you can be enthusiastic about what you know. Enthusiasm is infectious. Students want to learn from those who care. If we study and learn what is of interest to us, it translates more naturally into the hearts of our students. If you can say something from your heart because you understand it and care about it, it will land more fully with the student. Students want to connect to your experience and lessons and learn how to apply them to their lives.

BE A BEGINNER AGAIN

> *Your mind should be like an empty teacup. If it is already full, the universe*
> *can't fill it up. You must be open to receive, learn, and surrender.*
>
> ZEN PROVERB

Stay open to new ideas and new ways of expressing the old. If we listen to others with an open mind, we will learn something. Everyone has something to offer.

If we treat each pose, each class as if we had never been there before, we may learn something about ourselves. A habit mind is a closed mind.

CONTEMPLATE

The three stages of contemplation from Vedanta are ways in which we can turn knowledge into wisdom.

SHRAVANA—HEAR THE TRUTH

Traditionally, to learn the Sūtra (yoga verses written in Sanskrit) students would sit and chant. Without explanation or understanding, the first job was to absorb the sound into your body and know the verses from the inside out. Once you could recite them you could study and question the meaning of the Sūtra.

To the Western mind this can be a difficult practice as we feel the tendency to question everything that comes to us. We want to know why.

The practice of Shravana is one of stilling your internal and external questions and learning to listen. From this point of view we can learn to absorb and become more of the witness to life without trying to interpret meaning.

MANANA—REFLECT ON THE TRUTH

Once we have welcomed and attuned to the messages, our job is to contemplate, filter and discern. Which of them keep knocking on your door? These are the ones that will keep prodding you until you listen, in the hope that you will turn to them. Which of the messages invites you to go deeper, be brave, step out?

NIDIDHYASANA—LIVE AND BREATHE YOUR TRUTH

Through listening and contemplation we arrive at realisation. Do you have the willingness now to step up and be brave? To take action and move in the direction you are being called? This last action is the path of the hero.

BALANCE THE TEACHING STYLES OR METHODS

Become skilled at different approaches. When Krishna was counselling Arjuna in the *Bhagavad Gita*, Arjuna at first didn't quite get the message. So Krishna said, *try this way, Arjuna, or this way*. He repeated the same idea in new ways.

Learners who have a good sense of their body, like dancers or long-time practitioners of body movement, are often kinaesthetic learners. Most of us will need visual prompts, as well as aural; some will need touch, some imagery. Some of us will require multiple approaches.

In life, we have physical, mental, emotional, and spiritual needs. Consider various techniques or methodologies to balance and meet some or all of these needs in your class.

MEANING BEFORE DETAILS

When we give meaning before details, we help students understand why they are doing something. Presenting to a class what they are about to learn or study invests students' interest in the theme, intention, or outcome. For example, 'In today's class, we will work with creating both mobility and stability in the hip joint.' Or: '*Dharma* is often translated as "life purpose". Today, through a series of standing poses and a short meditation, we will explore what it means to be faithful to our calling.'

PRACTICE

Whatever we teach, if we don't practice it ourselves, we are not teaching, we are just transferring information. When we practice, we understand the subject on many levels, in our bodies, our minds, and our hearts. We know what it feels like not to practice, and we know the inherent joys as well as the obstacles when we do practice.

Practice turns any subject into the well-worn clothing of experience. When we teach from experience, it makes our job less stressful and more meaningful.

Each practice we do also unites us with the whole idea of what it means to practice, to dedicate ourselves to something, and this in itself is valuable teaching.

The brain is neuroplastic, meaning that it can rewire itself through repeated action or thought to produce new neural pathways. Showing up on our mats day after day, even if only for a short while, creates new grooves of seeing, being, and living.

Each time we show up to practice we receive alms for the heart, mind and body. The more we practice, the more these gifts will flood our outheld bowls. Each gift is a jewel not intended to be kept a secret, but instead to be offered back into the collective whole of our families, our communities and our classes.

BE CREATIVE AND TAKE RISKS

Creativity is our birthright; we were put on this planet to express ourselves. Being creative is using your imagination to bring something into being. This book contains lots of ideas to stimulate your imagination and bring inspiration to the forefront. Creativity is another expression of authenticity. Do you want to stand out or go with the crowd? Dare to dream and experiment with the limitless ways you can present your class. Be like the Queen of Hearts, who tells Alice in Wonderland to believe in six impossible things before breakfast. The yoga practice is a blank canvas. You get to create what you want.

LEAVE YOUR EGO AT THE DOOR

Your ego, as defined in yoga, is your belief system about yourself. *I am a good teacher; I am a bad teacher. I am good at yoga; I am bad at yoga. I know more than the students; I don't know enough. The class was good; the class was bad. The students like me; the students don't like me.*

All of these stories are just that—stories. They are personal constructs that take you further away from one of the definitions of yoga: that we are much more than who we think we are.

When you get yourself out of the way and leave your worries at the door you become a vessel for the teachings. You are there to serve and transmit your energy, love, and appreciation of whatever you teach. The students' needs should rise above your stories, even if just for this hour. Instead, when you walk into the room just bring these two things: your love of the practice and a willingness to serve. This will radiate into the energy of your teaching so everyone may benefit.

SEE AND HEAR, RECOGNISE AND APPRECIATE, ELEVATE AND EMPOWER

The secret in education lies in respecting the student.

RALPH WALDO EMERSON

Respect and understand the intelligence and potential of your students. You may have a beginner in body but not in mind. You may have someone struggling who is on the verge of a breakthrough. Remember, we don't know what path someone has walked before they come through the door.

Empower students. We are the caretakers of our students' hearts and minds. We get to touch others with words and movement that should usher people in the direction of elevation rather than towards fear.

DO YOU WANT TO BE A GOOD TEACHER OR A POPULAR TEACHER?

A good teacher is also a good leader. A leader will blaze paths, be okay with uncertainty, hold the unknown and the known in balance and teach from their hearts. A popular teacher teaches what they think is expected of them or what they think students want. When you decide to be a good teacher you will unburden yourself from the need to gain others' votes, you will strip yourself of the stress of having to be anything other than what you are. A good teacher is comfortable with losing students in order to gain the ones who are waiting for them. A good teacher knows who they are and what they want to offer.

THE LANGUAGE OF TEACHING

What doesn't add will subtract.

ARISTOTLE

We guide with our words. We can help heal, illuminate, and elevate—such is the power of language. When teaching, consider a choice of words that firstly instruct, secondly enrich, and thirdly empower.

Here are some points to consider for scripting yoga classes.

CHOOSE ESSENTIAL LANGUAGE

Less information is more powerful and lands with the student. Pauses give students a chance to breathe, feel, and embody the teachings. Consider this sentence:

'Instructionwordswordswordswordswordsagainoverandoveragaintalkingtalkingnonstop.'

The mind is not given space to absorb, so it tends to block all the words out and go into the thinking mind.

Students come to class from busy lives and situations that continually compete for their attention. This overabundance of stimuli means that we need to create an environment of space and peace so the practice can be absorbed rather than rejected.

YOU DON'T NEED TO BE PROFOUND

You need to be real, authentic, and understood. Choose clear, succinct language to convey your point.

USE BOTH ACTION CUES AND DESCRIPTIVE CUES

Compare the following cues:

> ACTION CUE
  Lift the four sides of your waist.

This type of cue gives the student a job to do or a task to complete, as opposed to describing what might be happening. Action cues are best to use when you want the student to get from A to B.

> DESCRIPTIVE CUE

The four sides of your waist lift.

This type of cue describes energy or passive movement. The students may listen but not do anything with their body. Descriptive cues are often more poetic and speak to the heart. These types of cue carry themes well.

Consider your cues to be giving directions to someone who is lost. They either want to be told how to get somewhere, or they want to be consoled or encouraged.

There is a time for both types of cues in your teaching.

AVOID FILLER WORDS AND/OR REPEATING THE SAME WORDS

We often use filler words such as 'nice' and 'good' without knowing it, to fill spaces while we think. Try being comfortable with spaces between cues and paring your language down to the essentials.

AVOID REPEATING THE SAME TYPE OF CUE OVER AND OVER

'Inhale and step your right leg forwards' could be:

Breathe in and step your right leg forwards.

Fill up and step your right leg forwards.

On your next breath in step your right leg forwards.

Take a full breath in and step your right leg forwards.

EXPERIMENT WITH LINKING TWO CUES TOGETHER

We can use the word *as* to link two cues together. Compare:

Root down into your feet. Lift your torso to the sky.

~with~

As you root down into your feet, feel your torso lift to the sky.

YOUR OR THE?

The word 'your' connects students to their body. Compare:

Step your right foot forwards.

  ~with~

Step the left foot forwards.

METAPHOR AND SIMILE

Metaphor and simile can bring music to the soul, as Voltaire wrote. Used sparingly, they are beautiful ways to help conjure up the beauty and grace of our bodies or to remind us of our interconnectedness with nature. Imagery taps students into the feeling or tone of the class and helps the practice become more somatic. It can transport students out of their head and into what is arising in their bodies.

METAPHOR

Metaphors are phrases that invoke imagery. These expressions refer to something that is not real, but we can imagine it to be so.

Your feet become the giant roots of a tree.

Feel your albatross wings spread wide.

Pour your breath into the container of your body.

SIMILE

A simile is a phrase that uses the words 'like' or 'as' to compare two seemingly unrelated things.

Feel your breath move in and out of you like a spring tide.

Soften the large muscles in your neck and shoulders as if they were butter melting.

CONSIDER THE LANGUAGE OF PERMISSION

Language of permission gives the students agency to make their own choices when practicing, and in doing so they become their own teachers. It is more inclusive to invite students into action, as it allows them to move within the parameters of their body on that day. It sets a tone in the class that they are safe to experiment with postures and adapt them to suit their needs.

Compare the more direct cues with the inviting cues:

DIRECT LANGUAGE	LANGUAGE OF PERMISSION
Take Child's pose	Feel free to take Child's pose if it is calling you
Move your torso to the right	Try moving your torso to the right and see how that makes the pose feel
If Crescent is too hard for you, drop your left knee to the floor	How does it feel to place one knee on the floor?
Lower level or beginner students do x	If it feels better, you could try this version
Skip the vinyasa if you need a rest	What feels most nourishing for you now?
After Kapalabhati you should feel y	Note what your experience of Kapalabhati is
If you can't do Pigeon, lay on your back and do x	Explore the alternatives for Pigeon
If you can't reach the ground, use a block	A block will bring the ground closer to your hand
Step your right foot to your right hand	Step your right foot in the direction of / towards your right hand
Step to the front of your mat	Hop, skip, dance or crawl to the front of your mat

MOVE YOUR LANGUAGE FROM FEAR-BASED TO FEELING-BASED

If we are told something may hurt or could cause us pain and that we need to be careful, then we are going to move our bodies as if we are fragile and should be fearful. This is known as the *Nocebo Effect*—any language that has a negative effect on our beliefs, as opposed to the *Placebo Effect*—language that has a positive effect on our beliefs.

NOCEBO	PLACEBO
Don't Don't crunch into your low back	Lengthen out of your low back to create spaciousness.
Never Never let your knee go over your ankle	Position your knee so it feels comfortable and supported.
Be careful of Be careful of straining your neck	Relax the large guy ropes of your neck.
Tight/stiff If you are tight in your hamstrings, bend your knees	Soften behind the backs of the knees to feel a release in your hamstrings.
Pain/painful You should put a bolster under your knee if it feels painful	I often use bolsters to support my knees in this pose.
Injured/injury Does anyone have any injuries I should be aware of?	Respect that all injuries are also a teacher. Find a way to love and support any parts of you that need special attention today.
Can/can't If you can't do Wheel then do Supported Bridge	One definition of an inversion is that you have your head below your heart. They all have the same benefits. Choose the variation of Wheel that is calling you today.
Watch (amazing student) do Wheel	Who here has not done Wheel before and would like to try?

Self-care

The yoga practice is like a salve or ointment,
a beautiful embodiment of self-care.

Before we begin teaching, we should consider if our own needs are being met. To serve, give, parent, teach, and respect others requires energy. It requires us to put on our own oxygen mask first. When we do this, we can give and live from a place of fullness.

We inhabit a busy world, and we can become overwhelmed in the body, heart, and mind. Fatigue and burnout can creep in if we are not in tune with our life. If we continually expend more energy than we acquire, we will move into depletion.

Self-care is not so much about a quick fix when life brings us to our knees. Self-care is an appraisal and acceptance of where we find ourselves at the moment.

To practice, we continually need to adjust our sails and gently nudge ourselves in the right direction. When we tend to ourselves in this way, we gently pull all our fragmented tendrils back home and put ourselves back together again.

Our body is the house for all of our experiences, so to understand ourselves more thoroughly, we need to take time to explore our home. Meeting yourself where you are daily, feeling into your body, and seeing what you have arrived with is the first step in embodied awareness.

SUFFER LESS

If you need to serve today, first serve yourself.

Buddhists describe suffering as an attachment to wanting things to be a certain way. Of course we want our classes to be outstanding and perfect, and wouldn't it be nice if we were praised or complimented? The truth is that people come to yoga for themselves, and the practice is not so much about you but the tools you present to help the students move towards a state of yoga.

We can't be responsible for how someone feels, acts, or interacts with us. We have no way of gauging what the student is thinking about us or the practice. There is definitely no chance of giving everyone what they want. We can't make them like us or like what we are teaching, nor should we try. It is quite possible we will forget a pose or the sequence and say things that make no sense. We will most likely leave out that stellar quote, approach someone who wants to be left alone, or ignore someone who wants to be seen. The music might be wrong, our voices not quite right. It's imperfect. It's cracked, flawed, and fissured.

What we *can* do is be a professional. Prepare yourself, prepare your class, and deliver it with authenticity and love. This is the medicine that will over time become the antidote that allays your fears. Then as the famous line in the *Bhagavad Gita* says: 'let go of the results.' The class finishes at the end when it finishes, not two hours later with the laments and should haves.

In the end, remember what Leonard Cohen sang to us:

Ring the bells that still can ring
Forget your perfect offering
There is a crack, a crack in everything
That's how the light gets in

POWERFUL MANTRA FOR THE TEACHER WITHIN

Like medicine, mantras can quickly shift our energetic state, neutralising our charge and making us a vessel for this thing we call yoga. Here is a selection of mantras to alleviate any tensions that you may have brought to the mat.

ARE YOU FEELING NERVOUS OR ANXIOUS?

Try a powerful standing pose, such as Warrior Two. Look down your front middle finger as if you are aiming. Feel your energy move from your head down into your heart.

Feel your feet and the sense of genuinely inhabiting your body.

Take a long slow breath in with the words '*I am committed*' and as you exhale, '*I choose to let go of doubt.*'

ARE YOU FEELING OVERWHELMED?

Try Humming Bee's Breath. Block off your ears, inhale, and as you exhale make a long, slow, high-pitch humming in the back of your throat. This bee-like sound drives out distractions and calms the mind. The long exhale activates the calming side of your nervous system.

Your mantra for overwhelm is '*Everything is going to be okay.*'

ARE YOU FEELING DISTRACTED?

If you feel distracted, try the Sa Ta Na Ma mantra. This mantra increases cognitive function and short-term memory. Tap the thumb to the index finger, *Sa*, to the middle finger, *Ta*, to the ring finger, *Na*, to the little finger, *Ma*. Repeat for at least three minutes.

Your mantra for distraction is '*Sa Ta Na Ma.*'

DO YOU FEEL LIKE YOU DON'T HAVE THE WORDS?

If you can't find your voice, try a round of *om*. *Om* stimulates the energy in the throat chakra through its vibration.

Your mantra to activate the power of your words is '*om.*'

DO YOU FEEL LIKE YOU HAVE IMPOSTER SYNDROME?

If you are having feelings of being a fraud—like you are faking it or you are not good enough to teach, remember a fraud is someone who is not being themselves. One beautiful set of words I was gifted when writing my first book was: '*Yes it's all been done before, yes there are better-qualified people with more experience, but they are not you, they don't have your voice.*' When you teach, be yourself.

Your mantra for these feelings is '*neti neti.*'

This mantra means *not this, not that.*

I am not this or that or who I identify myself to be. I am a spark of the divine.

DO YOU FEEL UNPREPARED TODAY?

The yoga poses are powerful medicine regardless of our words; they will work their magic. However, some days we may be late, feel unprepared, or show up and realise our plan is not going to land.

Walk into the room. Stand at the front and power up your legs—your roots into this ancient practice. Put the students in a pose. Breathe with them for five breaths.

Your mantra to prepare you is '*Everything is exactly as it is meant to be.*'

TEACHER RX

Wisdom is knowing I am nothing
Love is knowing I am everything
And between the two my life moves.

NISARGADATTA MAHARAJ

If you are to teach, you have to practice. When we learn through our bodies and minds, and we remain the ever-inquisitive student, we turn knowledge into wisdom. From teacher to student to teacher our life moves, and what flows from that is a transmission so fluid it is love itself.

The following practice is a simple sequence to stay connected to this flow.

HUG

Lay on your back with a bolster under your sacrum. Curl your knees into yourself. Feel how beautiful it is to be held.

When we learn to hold space for ourselves first, we are more able to do the same for others.

COMPASSION

Lie on your back with a bolster under your ribs and heart.
Remember what is important to you and why you teach.

Compassion is to emanate a presence so loving that when others shut down, turn away, or want to give up, we meet that with wanting to stay.

EARTHING

Come to a seat, join the soles of your feet together, and bow.
If you are fearful, ground yourself so that nothing can dislodge you.

Through your earthiness, you will be able to absorb and dissipate confusion or fear deep into the earth.

CONTAINER

Straighten out one leg, turn your ribs to the side, arch over your straight leg.
Feel into the boundaries of your side body.
Your insecurities may well up from your core as you prepare to teach.

When we welcome the fears, doubts, and insecurities arising within our container, it is the training in which we learn to do it for others.

THREE-PART BREATH

Inhale one-third of your breath; pause. Inhale to two-thirds full; pause. Inhale to the top of your breath, hold, and then slowly exhale.

The breath will fill you up and make energetic room to give.

SEATED MEDITATION

Find some way each day to observe yourself. Remind yourself that your noble job is to allow the teachings to live and evolve through you.

Mantra:

> *So Hum, I am that,*
> *Hum So, that I am.*

> *I am the universe, the universe*
> *I am*
> *I am that*
> *That I am*

Repeat this *So Hum* over and over, then sit in silence. Listen so profoundly it's as if you have put a shell to your ear and can hear into the chasm of the universe. Listen to the sweet messages she is sending to you today.

Care

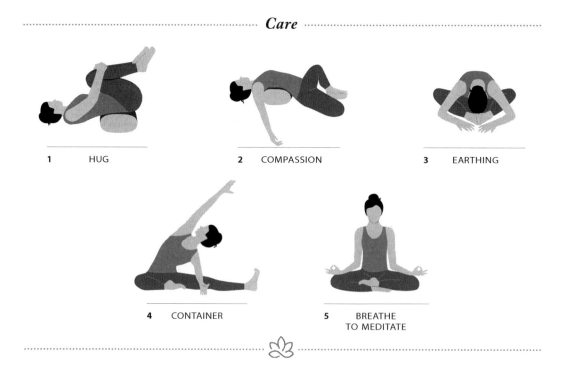

| 1 | HUG | 2 | COMPASSION | 3 | EARTHING |

| 4 | CONTAINER | 5 | BREATHE TO MEDITATE |

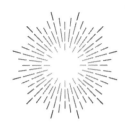

CHAPTER TWO

THE ART OF THEMING

WHAT IS A THEME?

A theme is the conversation we have during the poses that shines a light of awareness and intentionally magnifies one of the beautiful teachings implicit in yoga.

Themes are

+ a tapestry or sutra; many stitches woven together to form a picture.

+ conversations, questions or dialogues that provoke more profound thought or self-enquiry.

+ stories that convey meaning.

+ anything that you wish to shed light on or that you want to bring into awareness.

+ a way to embody the practice of life on and off the mat.

+ an enmeshment of life practice with yoga practice.

+ a tool to facilitate self-learning; deeper willingness and bravery to look at ourselves.

+ universal. (Intentions are personal promises. See 'Intend' for more information on setting intentions.)

WHY THEME?

Eventually, if we practise yoga for long enough, we will start to see that the postures, transitions, successes, and falls on the mat mirror an ordinary life. Themes issue an open invitation for students to unblur the lines between how they are on the mat and how they are in their lives.

Through intelligent theming, we gently open the doors to an individual's awareness of their actions and reactions, where they are holding on, their habit minds, and where they are stuck in their body or in their life.

Sensitive teachers guide students to form a more compassionate and observant relationship to themselves, while at the same time making them feel safe both physically and emotionally.

When we theme, we layer a richness into the practice. This gift will ultimately impel those who are curious to investigate more about what it means to be human, to love more fully, to let go of the unnecessary, and to uncover the beauty that lies within.

When used as a tool, themes

+ are a framework for the teacher to shape their class with.

+ give cohesion to a class.

+ provide a focal point, like a drishti, for both the teacher and student.

+ provide students with insight into the field of yoga and how it can apply to their life.

+ instil a more holistic understanding of yoga.

+ can remind the student of something they had forgotten.

+ are a way to bridge our own understanding of yoga into the lives and minds of the students.

Finding inspiration

We need inspiration to plan a class, which can be the most challenging part. Yoga is vast, and so we can enter into decision fatigue: with so many choices, where do we start? Here are some guidelines for streamlining your planning:

What are you working on in your spiritual practice?
Start there—at your most embodied understanding of yoga.

If you are working on stilling your mind or not getting caught up in dramas, note how that plays out for you in your life. What situations arise for you; how do you deal with them? When is it difficult, and when is it easy to follow your practice?

When you meet yourself *where* you are, you lessen the demand to be anything other than the rich theme of *who* you are. Investigations like this turn your classes into conversations and love letters from your heart.

Why do you teach yoga?
This question is critical: when you know *why* you are doing something, the *how* takes care of itself.

How do you define yoga?
There are as many definitions of yoga as there are yoga teachers. Your definition can be the driver behind the themes that feel soulful for you. If your definition of yoga is that it is a connection to all living beings, then your themes may reflect interconnection with nature.

Meditate
Sometimes our demand to find just the right theme can cloud thought processes. Meditation is a tool of solitude that lights up our prefrontal cortex like a Christmas tree. It takes us to the creative, decision-making parts of our mind and induces a calmness that ultimately makes things more transparent. Some of my best inspiration has come from slow walking or meditating.

When you sit, do so not to get the answer but to be open to what arises. Do it to clear a space for yourself and to listen.

No man ever steps in the same river twice,
for it's not the same river and he's not the same man.

HERACLITUS

Sit in nature

Nature offers rich and complex themes to braid through your class. Interconnection to the mystery and wonder of this planet can spark things within us. If we open our eyes to the world around us we will find inspiration. Stars and full moons, tides and birds, tiny bees, and plants growing are all our teachers. Contemplate the ways you can connect the most simple actions of nature to a life well lived.

Once you have chosen a theme you are interested in, teach from it for at least a week. Develop it by adding new information or reworking what you have already presented. Students will enjoy the repetition as they get to understand new concepts or philosophy of yoga. Every time you teach it will be a different river and you will be standing in a different place in your life.

INDUCING A THEME

We can look at the components of a yoga class—the asana, pranayama, mudra, etc.—and create our theme. An example of this would be to focus the class on forward folds and ask what themes arise for us while doing this group of postures. A folding theme may be introspection, honouring and respecting our past, or quieting the mind.

DEDUCING A THEME

Take the overall feeling, or *bhava* (feeling) wish to cultivate and work backwards.

An example could be that we want our class to feel balanced or equanimous. To tie this to our theme, we would look at the stitches we want to include. We may choose poses that challenge our balance, twists that look to both sides of life, or dive deeper into the meaning of *sthira* (strength) and *sukha* (ease).

STREAMLINE YOUR PLANNING

Here is a guide to the nuts and bolts of writing your theme.

✦ Decide on a theme of interest to you, e.g. the first chakra.

Choose one chakra. You could also decide on your group of poses or peak pose and decide which chakra works best with your choice.

✦ Brainstorm what you already know about the theme.

Have a general understanding of the chakra system but have more specific information on the chakra you have chosen.

✦ Connect your theme to the yoga of (your) life.

How does the theme you have chosen relate to your life? How could it relate to the people in your class? What do you want the students to take home with them? For example, '*The first chakra relates to our place on the earth and being grounded.*'

✦ Connect your theme to yoga philosophy.

How does your chosen theme intersect with the wisdom from the *Yoga Sūtra*, the *Bhagavad Gita*, or the *Tao Te Ching*? Any teaching that examines the nature of life and our existence makes for rich fodder to layer into your theme.

✦ Connect your theme to asana.

Which poses embody the theme? The first chakra relates to our feet, legs, and connection of the legs into the pelvis. Do you want to heat and generate strength and stability in these parts of the body, or do you want to open and release?

✦ Start teaching the theme from the first pose.

Pick warm-ups and cues that work directly with or bring awareness to the feet. For example, '*Press the tops of your feet down in Upward Facing Dog.*' In the body of the class, start to build heat for the peak pose/s or sequence/s. Select cool-down poses to balance, open, and counter the theme and the body.

✦ Consider the energy curve to your class.

Every class has one or more energy curves. The most common is the bell curve. Much like the *trimurti* (Brahma to create, Vishnu to maintain, and Shiva to dissolve), the class will have a natural beginning, peak, and end. Such a curve might look like this:

- Warm-ups: setting intentions, opening quote or statement, opening postures, Sun Salutations
- Body of class: standing poses, peak poses or peak sequences
- Cool-downs: floor poses, closing poses
- Finishing: blessings, quotes, gratitude

✦ Decide on your bhava.

Bhava means the feel, emotion, or tone of the class. Do you want the students to feel relaxed or powerful and strong?

✦ What actions embody the theme?

For the first chakra, you might consider using the action of rooting down into the feet. In other classes, you may concentrate on spiralling, lifting, expansion, or contraction.

✦ Encapsulate your theme in a few key statements.

For example, '*The chakras line the spine and are represented as spinning wheels of energy. Each chakra is thought to develop at a specific phase of our life, and they all represent a different quality. The yogis who mapped these energy centres believed that good health relied on the quality of energy at each chakra.*'

Or: '*We will embody the theme of the first chakra by working with our feet, legs, and our foundations.*'

✦ Collect supportive words and phrases and creative imagery.

Use a thesaurus to collect words, synonyms, antonyms, and word origins.

For example, chakra: wheel, spinning, orb, vortex, energy, prana, qi, roots, family, belonging.

✦ Gather inspirational readings and quotes.

Using the first chakra as an example, quotes and readings that encapsulate the earth, grounding, roots, feet, and stability will bring a flourish to your class.

✦ Consider choosing a pranayama practice.

We cleanse the nervous system and the mind and open up energy channels through pranayama. How will you instruct the breath and tie it into the theme?

For the first chakra, consider pranayama that is grounding.

✦ Use the tools of meditation and mudra to link to your theme.

With the first chakra, consider using mudras that are earthy, such as Prithvi mudra (join the thumb to the tip of the earth or ring finger), which promotes a feeling of stability, security, and strength.

SHARING FROM YOUR LIFE

Themes that arise in our life, our struggles and successes, our heartbreaks and joys, are part of living in these bodies. Here are some things to consider when sharing personal themes:

If the students don't know you or haven't built a relationship with you, personal themes may not land as well. An out-of-context life theme will seem irrelevant to their worlds.

Students can be genuinely curious about their teacher, so a story about something you are going through will help them realise that we are all in this together. However, in theming your class, always find a way to connect the dots of your life to their lives.

If what you are experiencing now has not been fully digested and worked through in your life, it may not be a good time to share it. Share the universal teachings of personal stories rather than the unprocessed rawness of what you may be experiencing. We have to walk through our challenges to understand the teachings or lessons behind them. This is when we see the jewels of heartbreaks, lessons, and learnings.

As you work through your situation, what tools or solutions from the yogic teachings apply to you, or have you found useful? Your teaching will become more potent if you can relate the problem to the tools to the teaching, giving your students a powerful recipe for change.

Leaving students with a takeaway or homework allows them to develop the theme further in their own lives.

Dharma diving

Dharma talks, taken from the Buddhist tradition, convey teachings through story, anecdote, and wise words, and are a powerful way to set the vision for your class.

Any life experience, yoga or life philosophy, personal story, reading, or quote can form the basis and inspiration for your talk. Your life is the imperfect perfect ground from which to teach. The problems and the triumphs that you have are reflected like a hall of mirrors onto all of our lives. The fissures and flaws in your human experience are an opening to awareness of life's duality.

Here are some guidelines for diving into dharma:

+ Dharma talks should be under two minutes for a sixty-minute class.

+ They should be at the start of class but can come after one posture or meditation. Sometimes we need to go through the body to get to the heart.

+ They can be based on a quote, a poem, yoga philosophy, an event in your life, or an emotion like love, patience, or gratitude.

+ The key teaching should be expanded on in the middle and towards the end of the class, like a dharma sandwich.

+ Use essential, coherent language to convey your point.

+ Tie your talk to the philosophy of yoga and the physical practice. This helps the lessons steep and gain magnitude.

+ Make your personal story universal so students can relate to it. It should meet the needs of the listener and be relevant to them.

+ Your anecdotes should be authentic. You should have experienced them and understood them in your life.

+ Don't be afraid to repeat your main point in many different ways. Think about digging a deeper hole as you progress in the class. If we take too many detours with our message, it gets diluted.

+ Listen to dharma talks. Try Jack Kornfield, Tara Brach, and Michael Stone for inspiration, stories, and wisdom.

+ Be consistent. If you want to do dharma talks, give them in most or all classes. Students will know what to expect from you, and the talks will become a more natural part of your teaching.

ONE-MINUTE THEMING

Sometimes all we need is a shot of inspiration to take into our class. These one minute wonders are tried and true and you will find some of them in more detail in the book.

Yoga philosophy as a teaching

When you change your breath, you change everything.

It is possible to be kind all the time, especially to yourself.

It's okay to mess things up, it's okay to fall over, it's okay to start again.

We are all connected.

Live and speak your truth.

The goal is balance.

How we do anything is how we do everything.

It is possible to change things.

Everything changes, nothing is permanent.

Letting go is the key.

It's not how it looks, it's how it feels.

Forgiveness is medicine for happiness.

We are not in control.

Love trumps fear.

Get to know yourself a little better.

Stop trying so hard.

Slow down a little.

The body can only heal in stillness.

Faith is an understanding that things are going to work out precisely in the right way for you.

Follow your dreams.

You are stronger than you think.

Your body is smarter than your brain.

What challenges you, changes you.

Whatever we resist, persists.

Setting an intention is the seed for all change.

You can choose to react or respond to your life.

It's okay to feel stuff.

Every body is different. Everybody is different.

Have the courage to be yourself.

Build your house on a rock.

Agreeing with life takes less effort than moving against it.

P is for practice, not perfection.

Yoga defined

Yoga is an art and a science.

Yoga is a technology that helps us connect to the part of us that is unspoilt, the place that can never be hurt or damaged.

The practice of yoga helps us step out of our comfort zone and habits.

If it doesn't change you, it isn't yoga.

Yoga gives us a unique pattern of movements to take us from the ordinary to the extraordinary.

Yoga transforms our world and how we see it, even if it's just for this hour.

Yoga is breath.

Yoga teaches us to coexist with all parts of ourselves.

Yoga is a conversation we have with ourself.

Yoga is the science of relationships.

Yoga is a practice.

Yoga is unity with ourselves, with others, and with the environment.

Yoga is the practice of living in alignment with our life.

One-word themes

Non-attachment

Non-judgement

Letting go

Quieting and stilling

Peacefulness

Beginner's mind

Gratitude

Surrender

Love, devotion, and service

Compassion

Commitment

Balance

Wisdom

Presence

OTHER CONSIDERATIONS

Believe in yourself. Trust that you have something to share. Your life is unique.

Trust your instincts. There will be a perfect time to share, so learn to listen to when that moment is and when it isn't.

Each class is a live performance; you can't stop the tape and rewind. So be okay when you 'trip up' and keep moving on.

Not everything you say is going to land beautifully; this is the price you pay for stepping out of your comfort zone.

At the end of class, resist the phone call to the judges of your mind.

There are some things that don't always land well:

+ Oversharing or talking too much.

+ Unrelated or random nuggets. It's better to create a container for your theme and stick with it.

+ Imparting complex themes while the student is struggling with a pose. The mind can usually only deal with one complexity at a time.

+ Switching quickly between philosophy and instructions. Imparting a nugget of philosophy followed immediately by 'now step your left leg through' doesn't give students time to digest either the words of wisdom or the cue.

+ Using a theme like joy, happiness, or gratitude without mentioning its opposite. These bright shiny themes only exist because of their opposite. Exploring opposite states gives a richness to what we are trying to impart. It also helps more students connect to the theme. If your theme is gratitude and a student already feels grateful, they may switch off to your message. However, mentioning the amnesia and complacency we can all suffer when we take our lives for granted serves as a reminder.

The word 'happiness' would lose its meaning
if it were not balanced by sadness.

CARL JUNG

FINAL THOUGHTS

Questions inspire thought and creativity in the receiver. They also create a natural pause time in which students can consider what the question means to them. Questions open situations up; statements can close things down.

Don't assume you know the effect of your words. Words carry energy and potency that lingers long after you have spoken. Your words might not be 'heard' by everyone, but if it lands with just one person that is enough. In some of my classes I have felt that students were uninterested in what I had to say. Then I would walk out, and a student would comment, '*I needed to hear that.*'

Realise that the experience the students are having will differ from student to student, and vastly differ from what you are experiencing. When we understand that, we can lighten up on how someone feels or reacts to our classes. Sometimes the 'worst' class we teach can be the best class for someone else. Sometimes we think we have done our best work and everyone walks out without a word.

Some days will be tough. We can't 'control-alt-delete' our performances; we may feel disconnected to what we are doing, or out of sync with the students. We may be a substitute teacher for someone who is 'popular'; we may feel unwell or unprepared. On these days, rely on the less-is-more approach and let the postures of yoga speak for themselves.

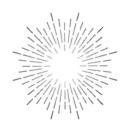

CHAPTER THREE

SOUL-FULL STARTS

Temporal landmarks are moments in time where we get to wipe the slate clean and start again. These fresh starts happen at significant life events, the beginnings of days, weeks, or years, and when we lay down our mat and roll it back up. New beginnings open our minds to change and possibility, making us receptive to ideas.

The dawn of a class is the perfect time to plant the seeds for what is about to arise.

We can begin our classes

- ✦ in a posture
- ✦ with pranayama
- ✦ with mantra or chanting
- ✦ with story, words, quotes, or dharma talks

The following ideas and practices are perfect ways to highlight the importance and potency of new beginnings.

INTEND

Once you make a decision, the universe conspires to make it happen.

RALPH WALDO EMERSON

San: true

Kalpa: a rule that is above all rules

Sankalpa: heartfelt intention

Themes: attention, intention, alignment, new year

We are born with the energy to create, the power to love without condition, and the strength to overcome our obstacles. Sankalpa helps us uncover our inherent goodness and our natural talents and unfold them out into the world.

Sankalpa can be something you want to bring into your life, to create or manifest, or it could be an inherent value you would like to embody. When we set this promise for a day, for one project, for a lifetime, or for the beginning of something important, we create a will to stay true and connected to that task. As humans, we are filled to the brim with desires. Sankalpa acts as a divining rod to direct our will to those desires that are purposeful and will bear fruit.

The quality of your life is determined by how much energy, interest, and attention you bring to it and how willing you are to act in alignment with your heart's desires. Do you know what you want for your life? Do you know how you want to feel or be? Our purpose in life is to find meaning and give our energy and devotion to that.

Be willing to hear the desires of your heart.
Be willing to support your intention.
Be willing to respond to the call of action.

Sankalpa takes a different approach to resolutions, which tend to dissolve quickly into the background. It understands that you are already whole, you have all that you need, and your wish is not coming from a place of lack.

THE PRACTICE

Ask the questions you have welling up within to help you find your sankalpa—your highest intention for this day, this life. Every question is a chance to take a personal inventory and to help bring clarity and focus to your core values.

We can ask ourselves

What qualities would I like to embody today?

What is tapping on my heart?

What is it that I want to achieve in this life?

What is important to me?

What or who do I value?

What am I tired of learning?

What are my reactive patterns when life challenges me?

And if you are stuck, ask yourself, 'Which of the divine qualities of the heart are calling me?'

❧ *Divine Qualities of the Heart* ☙

bliss	clarity
peace	purity
harmony	unity
love	compassion
understanding	kindness
empathy	forgiveness

When you have your answer, set your intention as a succinct, present tense, positive statement, such as:

I follow my dreams.

I am loved.

I am patient.

I am kind.

I have all I need to live a full life.

I feel calm when life is hectic.

I manage my time well.

MORNING SANKALPA MEDITATION

We are born with Buddha nature, so there is no need to fix anything but rather to reveal the parts that have been covered over. This meditation helps access this part of you, and from there find your sankalpa.

To access our sankalpa, we need to get quiet and to go beyond the conscious brain.

Today we will uncover the part of you that wants to be seen and heard, that is already there, just waiting for your attention.

So, take your seat, get quiet and comfortable. Relax your shoulders, your face, and let your hips be heavy to the earth.

Turn your right hand palm-up on your right thigh.

Turn your left palm up in line with your heart.

Rock your left hand across your heart, like you are rocking a baby.

Swim your hand across the current of your heart.

Cradle your heart's desires.

Now place your left palm face-up on your right palm.

This is Sankalpa mudra.

Close your eyes, soften the outwards gaze, turning your sight inwards, towards your heart.

Soften the space between the eyes all the way back to the spot in the centre of the brain, the third eye, the seat of all-knowing.

Draw the breath in from both nostrils and feel the convergence at the midbrain, as if two streams become one.

See a soft light here; the yogis call this light jyoti, the supreme radiance within.

Let this light soothe your midbrain.

Feel the light expand, and as if you were swallowing it whole, take it to your heart and let it fill up this area.

Listen.

What is the message you receive?

Find a secret place to hold the words in your heart and repeat them daily. When we set our sankalpa each daybreak, we bring more focus, more attention to what it is we need to achieve and thereby redirect our energy to where it needs to go.

Things will shift for you slowly. The intention will take form as we set it into action with our words, deeds, and thoughts.

Be there to see the change.

Offer

Even after all this time, the sun never says to the earth, you owe me.
Look what happens with a love like that, it lights the whole sky.

Hafiz

Anjali: divine offering

Themes: living your life as an offering, letting go, interconnection

In Balinese culture, at the break of day you can smell incense weave through the air. Locals gather at the sea and villages to make offerings to the gods with flowers, fruit, and biscuits placed with love on the sand or ground. These hallowed offerings are placed with reverence. Each flower is carefully chosen for its colour and arranged as a gift to a different deity. Their offerings are to appease, offer thanks, and bless, but also to remember that we are part of an intricate network of support. A loving symbiotic relationship means to give as well as receive.

As the days wear on, the offerings are carried away by the tide, trampled on, or eaten by stray animals. No one mourns their demise as the power in the offering is also in the letting go.

Make your practice an offering.

There are two ways we can experience yoga and ultimately our lives. We can do it as if everyone owes us and we need to get something out of it, or we can do it with love and in service.

When you are on your mat, consider offering your practice to someone in need, someone you love, or even to someone who you feel 'owes' you or doesn't deserve your full love and affection. When we practice through the lens of giving and serving without expectation, we can subtly shift our consciousness from lack to fullness. This generosity is a self-replicating gift. We may not see the brightness of our work, but someone, somewhere will.

This is how we light the sky up every day.

THE PRACTICE

❧ *Anjali Mudra Offering* ☙

This symbol of connection joins the left and the right hemispheres of the brain, forming balance and establishing concentration.

Lean your hands into each other like an angel's wings.

When we join our palms together like this, we are not praying but offering.

We are not asking but giving.

Raise your hands high above your head.

We offer this practice up to all those who have come before us, our teachers, our lineage, our ancestors. It is through this gesture that we connect and honour and show gratitude to all who have walked this path. We offer up what concerns us so that we may be free of attachment.

Bring your hands to your third eye centre.

We offer this practice to the wisdom of life. May all those who seek guidance, understanding, and clarity find what they are searching for.

Bring your hands to your lips.

We offer this practice to the sweetness of all of our words, both spoken and written. May we remember that through the power of speech, we can hurt or heal, give or take away.

Bring your hands to your heart.

We offer this practice to the well-being of all souls who need security, love, food, care, and companionship. May this gesture remind us of how much we have, how connected we are, and of the abundance of life.

Anjali Mudra Flow

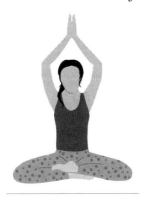

1   ANJALI MUDRA

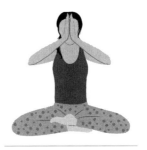

2   ANJALI MUDRA
AT THE FOREHEAD

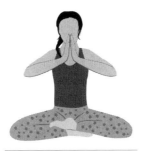

3   ANJALI MUDRA
AT THE MOUTH

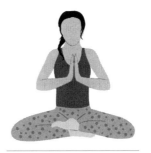

4   ANJALI MUDRA
AT THE HEART

Vow

Love is composed of a single soul inhabiting two bodies.

ARISTOTLE

Bodhi: being

Sattva: enlightenment

Bodhisattva: a spiritual practitioner who devotes their life to service and awakening

Theme: wherever you put your attention or energy will grow and flourish

Patanjali tells us in the *Yoga Sūtra* that if we want to be successful at yoga, the practice must be steady and consistent, performed over time and done with love. Yoga is ultimately a lifelong tool to foster steadiness in our life and thoughts. We cultivate our capacity for holding all of life by showing up.

We show up in some way every day because we realise the pain of not practising is louder than any pain the practice may bring.

THE PRACTICE

I am the bodhisattva of my life, a noble and awakened heart.

In the Buddhist tradition, the bodhisattva is an enthusiastic spiritual practitioner who is willing to make an effort over a long period to achieve spiritual awakening. They do this for the good of themselves but also for the love of all sentient beings. Their path covers decades of work and hundreds of miles without cessation to carry the torch of happiness and well-being for us all.

I vow to show up

Often people question how to practice. Should I practice in the morning or evening? How long should I practice? What technique is best? What if I miss a practice? The most crucial moment of any practice is to arrive, to seal the intention to bring the practice to life. All the rest is commentary.

I vow to share

When we finish our yoga or meditation, we must harness the goodness that we have uncovered and offer it into the world as a radical presence.

There is no point doing yoga, meditation, or spiritual practice if you keep the jewels for yourself.

No person or corner of your life should be excluded from this beautiful awareness you create.

We all have a role in the collective puzzle to play. Through sharing, we ensure the practice stays alive in the collective hearts and minds.

I vow to notice

The last, most important part of any practice is realising.

The practice is a tool for cultivating qualities of peace, faith, love, and patience.

The benefits of any practice will show up unannounced when you least expect them but when you most need them.

Maybe you notice that you are less reactive, you feel more grounded and fulfilled, or you begin to like yourself more.

Maybe you notice your life is better in some way.

Maybe you notice in the most difficult or suffocating moment a sense of freedom.

Tick them off; they are signs of your evolution.

Bodhisattva

Take your seat, be at ease.

Thank yourself for taking the time to show up and to practice.

Whatever you commit to, wherever you put your energy, will flourish.

Like any relationship, be it yoga practice, a marriage, a business, if it is to grow, there has to be a commitment.

Bring your hands to your heart.

Bow your head in appreciation of these commitments you have made to yourself and others.

I am the bodhisattva of my life, a noble and awakened heart.

I vow to show up.

I vow to share.

I vow to notice.

May this practice fall like a snowflake into the hearts and minds of those in need.

SING

A rising tide lifts all boats.

UNKNOWN

Sangha: community

Themes: interconnection, empowerment, community, study and learning

The Blue Zone is a triangle of five regions linked by the longevity of their citizens. They are Okinawa (Japan), Sardinia (Italy), Nicoya (Costa Rica), Icaria (Greece), and Loma Lina (California). Studies have been done to understand why the inhabitants lead such long and healthy lives. Besides moving their bodies and eating a mainly plant-based diet, the residents actively participate in their community, know others' names, stand by, help each other when needed, and put family above everything else. More importantly, their life is led by a sense of purpose and meaning that they gain from caring, helping, and watching out for others[2]. The Okinawans call this *ikigai;* the yogis call it *sangha.*

We may have all come in different ships, but we're in the same boat now.

MARTIN LUTHER KING, JR.

In yoga, sangha means community. When we practice together, we gain strength from each other. When we have a sense of belonging in a group, we empower ourselves and others. We understand the responsibility of a group: to uphold the structure with tender love and care. When we assemble for a single purpose, united in our beliefs, we climb higher.

Sanskrit is a vibrational language; the letters and syllables carry a resonance that once uttered or sung passes energy through you and out into the world. To understand the word is to understand its significance. Traditionally learnt through call and response, the mantra below whispers to us: *connection, community* and *learning.*

---

[2] Dan Buettner, *The Blue Zone Kitchens.* (National Geographic, 2019).

THE PRACTICE

❧ *Shanti Mantra* ❧

Man: mind, derived from the word *man*—'to think'

Tra: vehicle or tool

Mantra: a sacred tool to help the mind cross over from mental clutter to mental clarity

> Om Saha Nau
> Om Saha nau vavatu
> Saha nau bhunaktu
> Saha viryam karavavahai
> Tejas vi navadhi tamastu
> Ma vidvisavahai
> Om Shanti, Shanti, Shanti

Om

Let us come together to be protected and nourished by the energy of the teachings
through the spirit of our understanding.

When we learn and practice together, we gain a strength that benefits
all of humanity and brings purpose to the paths we tread,
diluting our anger,
bringing peace and serenity
for us,
for nature,
for the divine.
Om peace, peace, peace.

TRANSITION

Every moment is a new beginning.

T.S. ELIOT

Nyasa: to place (your attention) at specific points of energy

Vi: in a special way

Krama: steps

Vinyasa krama: logical and progressive steps on the path building from the simple to the complex

Theme: our life is a vinyasa; transitions; change

Vinyasa is to place your body, breath, and mind with reverence in all of the poses. It is the mindful way we attend to each breath, each movement, and each thought. To dance with the current of life, to transition with grace, to breathe and move with whatever is arising, to be present and to work with difficulties and joys, is the true definition of vinyasa.

The two most important transitions we will make are the one into our life and the one out. All of the other moments, both welcome and not, stitch together to form the vinyasa of our lives. Like Brahma, Vishnu, and Shiva, every posture of life has a beginning, a middle, and an end—a birth, a life, and a death. Life becomes the bridge between our first inhale and our last exhale, joining all the dots, all the events into one long dance.

The life vinyasa is a process, a series of comings and goings, breaking down and building up, fruition and dissolution. To have the willingness to take part in it, breath by breath, moment by moment, movement by movement is an act of bravery. Life is challenging and unique; it holds no promises or guarantees, nor does it move how we demand it should. It is neither a puzzle to solve nor a problem to be fixed. It is a creative, unfolding process. Some transitions are sweet, some a little clunky. Some (life) poses we want out of, some we don't want to leave.

How you say goodbye, end a pose, leave a job, finish a class, or end a relationship carries energy into the next. Each thought, each breath, each action leads to another. The trick is to know and appreciate when something has finished, and transition with grace. If we cling to what has been, even when we know it is over, we leave no room for the new.

THE PRACTICE

Take your seat.

Flood your body with the breath.

Find stillness.

Get quiet.

Can you hear the vinyasa of your heart?

Its morse code is urging you to pay attention.

The energy you bring into this moment is the seed that will fill your practice.

Today, watch your transitions, how you enter and how you leave a pose—as we flow, move, and breathe together.

For how you do anything is how you do everything.

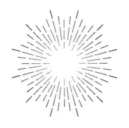

CHAPTER FOUR

SETTING FOUNDATIONS

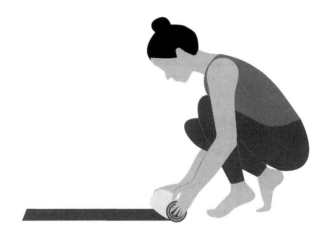

Do you wish to rise? Begin by descending.
You plan a tower that will pierce the clouds?
Lay first the foundation of humility.

SAINT AUGUSTINE

For us to be committed to anything in life, we need to fortify our foundations. In yoga we often say everything that touches the ground is our foundation, be it our hands, head, feet, or belly. We must learn to place the body in a way that unites us with the primary foundation of the earth and respects our physical support systems. From a strong foundation, we can ascend with grace and resilience.

Later, as we progress in our practice (once we have set our body foundations), we will need to consider the bedrock of our breath and the underpinnings of our mind and heart.

BODY SCAN PRACTICE

As above, so below, as within, so without, as the universe, so the soul.

HERMES TRISMEGISTUS

In our busy and at times distracted lives, we sooner or later take a vacation from our bodies and our attention drifts. Starting any class with a simple body scan will help reel back in all the parts of ourselves we gave away.

BODY TEMPLE

Find a comfortable seat where you are relaxed, at ease.

Inhale, lift your shoulders around your ears, and with a strong exhale, let them drop heavily.
Do this twice more. Lift and drop the shoulders, letting out a HA sound on your exhale.

Start by feeling into your body.
Like a bee investigating its flowers, flutter your attention from one body part to the next, looking for the sweetness in each.
There is no need to change anything as nothing is broken.
Instead, notice how each part feels.

Bring your attention to just above your head. Can you feel sensation there?
What do you perceive?

Sense your face, trace the bony landmarks,
the cheekbones,
jaw,
the rims of the eyes,
and the soft fleshy parts of your cheeks, lips, and ears.

Feel into the width of your shoulders.
Sense into the triangle of collarbones, sternum, and shoulder blades. Feel your shoulders drape, as though over a coat hanger.

Touch into the solar system of your belly,
your hips,
and into the long bones of your legs,
your feet and toes.

Become aware of your breathing.
Your breath is your energetic support system that feeds and nourishes you.
How are you feeding yourself?

What is your energy state?
Do you feel empty or full? Alert or tired?

To the mind now.
Note the mind, doing its job, carrying its hitchhiker thoughts.
What is going for a ride with you on your mat?
What wants to be heard or seen?

Note all of this with loving awareness.

When you are ready, rub your hands together, place them over your eyes. Feel the heat from your hands as you softly open your eyes.

PADA BANDHA

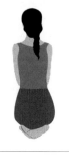

SWEET FEET

Walk as if you were kissing the earth with your feet.
THICH NHAT HANH

To the Mind

Pada: feet

Bandha: lock, tether, fasten

Themes: first chakra, grounding, stability, resiliency

LANGUAGE OF THE FEET

Feel lights in your heels

Spread and widen your feet like giant leaves

Feel the bones of the toes settle like small pebbles

Clip your weight evenly into the horseshoe of your heel

As you press down, feel a buoyancy in your foundations

Lay your weight evenly into the saddle of the heel bone

Feel the resiliency at the base of your foot like a trampoline

Imagine a secret flower under the instep of your foot that you don't want to crush

Lift up through the arches as if you were trying to pull energy up into your legs

Imagine your feet are like pumps, drawing goodness from the earth and pulling it up into your legs and pelvis

To the Heart

For us to feel stable while standing, we need a good base. Like a human horseshoe, the mound under the big toe, the mound under the little toe, and the centre of the heel make up a trident and reference points for us to kiss the earth. When we apply a downwards pressure to these three points, we are able to get heavy into the ground but feel a rebounding through the arches of the feet up into the body. Imagine standing in a lift: you can feel weighted, but you are also ascending. The lift of the arches and the centre of the foot, while pressing the horseshoe down, is known as *pada bandha*.

The blueprint of your whole body is reflected in your feet. According to reflexologists, areas of the feet reflect areas of the body. Look at your medial arch; it takes the shape of your spine. The sole of the foot is home for your organs, whereas the toes house the senses and the pineal and pituitary glands. Therefore, when we work the feet, we work the foundation of the whole body.

To the Body

❧ *Sweet Feet* ☙

Our feet are home to some of the thickest fascia in the body, known as the plantar fascia.

This practice works at creating a resiliency in the feet. A strong foundation is not a rigid one but one that can adapt to the changing needs of the structure.

TOE MASSAGE

1. Sit on the floor and cross your right ankle over your left thigh.

2. Interlace your right fingers between your toes.

3. Using your hand and ankle, make these movements: circle the ankle, flex and point the toes, squeeze the toes, and turn the foot upwards and downwards.

4. Repeat on the other side.

TOE LOCK

1. Interlace the toes of your left and right feet one by one as if you were knitting them together. This encourages spreading of the toes, which you can also focus on in standing poses.

BROKEN TOE

1. Start in Child's pose with your toes tucked under. This may be enough for some students. Gradually walk the hands back until you are sitting up with your shoulders over your hips. Stop prior to that if you feel a stretch in your toes.

2. Stay here for one minute.

TOE RELEASE

1. Lean forwards, untuck your toes, and roll back onto the tops of your feet.

INSTEP MASSAGE

1. Kneel.

2. Place the top of your right foot into the arch of your left foot.

3. Keep your hands on the ground or sit onto your heels for more intensity.

4. Repeat on the other side.

FOOT MASSAGE

1. Stand in Mountain pose.

2. Place a tennis ball or myofascial release ball under the sole of your right foot.

3. Roll the ball up and down your foot.

4. Apply enough pressure to feel mild to moderate sensation.

5. Repeat on the left side.

Sweet Feet

| 1 TOE MASSAGE | 2 TOE LOCK | 3 BROKEN TOE |
| 4 TOE RELEASE | 5 INSTEP MASSAGE | 6 FOOT MASSAGE |

Teaching Notes

+ Demonstrate the three mounds or the trident: under the big toe, under the little toe, and the centre of the heel, plus the arches (especially the medial arch). This can be done while sitting and further illustrated in standing poses.

+ In balancing poses, encourage a rebounding lift in the arches and a spreading but not gripping of the toes.

+ Walking meditations are a respectful way to bring mindful energy to the feet.

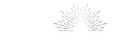

Hasta Bandha

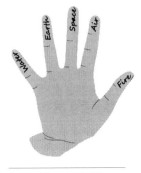

HASTA BANDHA

As you grow older you will discover that you have two hands,
one for helping yourself, the other for helping others.
Audrey Hepburn

To the Mind

Hasta: hand

Bandha: lock, tether, fasten

Themes: your life is in your hands, individuality, your uniqueness

LANGUAGE OF THE HANDS

Flare the fingers
Spread your hands like starfish
Claw the floor with your fingertips
Let your fingers reach out like quills
Hollow through the centre of your palms
Weave/interlace/intwine your fingers together
Press your palms together like two soft cloths
Feel energy spread out from the end of your fingers into infinity
As you lie in Savasana let the fingers furl of their own accord

To the Heart

The human hand and its twenty-seven bones hold the unique story of our lives, written on our palms. Anytime we place our hands on the earth we are entrusting our personal DNA to the support of the ground. They are the perfect tool, just the right shape, softness, and texture to hold on and let go, to serve and receive, to throw and catch. Just the right warmth and softness to hold the hand of someone in need.

To the Body

❧ *Wrist and Hand* ☙

When we bear weight on our hands, especially during vinyasa-style flows, we are asking the wrists and hands to support us. Overuse, collapsing into the wrist crease, and not engaging the muscles of the forearm can lead to injury.

The following practice is to bring awareness to the wrists and hands in preparation for arm balancing.

MUKULA MUDRA

1. Join your four fingers to your thumb to create a 'beak' shape.
2. Hold your arms at shoulder height out in front of you.
3. Turn and flex your wrists towards the earth.
4. Hold the mudra as you lift and lower your 'beak' by flexing and extending your wrists as if they were nodding yes.

WEB STRETCH

1. Hold your right hand out in front of you with your palm up at waist height; relax your elbow.
2. Grip your right thumb with your left hand and gently pull your thumb away from your fingers, then release.
3. Use your left hand to grip your little finger. Gently pull your little finger downwards. Release.
4. Repeat with your ring finger, middle finger, and index finger.
5. Change sides.

HIGH FIVE FLICK

1. Bring your hands to shoulder height with your palms facing outwards and your hands clenched.
2. Flick open your fingers.
3. Clench your fingers.
4. Repeat these two movements in a steady tempo for at least a minute.

WRIST SHIFTS

1. Come to Tabletop pose on all fours with your hands on the floor below your chest.

2. Turn your fingers out like starfish.

3. Make circular clockwise then anticlockwise movements with your body.

PALM AND FOREARM MYOFASCIAL RELEASE (MFR)

1. Come to Child's pose but lift your hips up a little.

2. Place your right hand on the floor, palm up.

3. Plant your left elbow in the middle of your right palm, with the left forearm standing upright.

4. Press down into the centre of the palm and move your left elbow in small circles.

5. Lay your right forearm on the ground completely from the elbow to the wrist.

6. Place your left forearm near your elbow crease so your foreams form a 'v' shape and apply pressure.

7. Move your left forearm down your right forearm until you reach the wrist. Linger at any point that feels tight.

GORILLA

1. Come to stand in Forward Fold.

2. Turn your palms upwards and inwards.

3. Lift up your feet and snuggle your hands under your feet. See if you can get the wrist crease to kiss the toes. Bend your knees as much as you need to.

4. Press down with your feet into the palms of your hands.

5. Move your weight forwards and back.

Wrist and Hand

1 MUKULA MUDRA

2 WEB STRETCH

3 HIGH FIVE FLICK

4 WRIST SHIFTS

5 PALM MASSAGE MFR

6 FOREARM MFR

7 GORILLA

Teaching Notes

HASTA BANDHA

The powerful *hasta bandha*, or hand lock, helps tone and lift the body away from the forces of gravity, creating a strength in our foundation and a lightness in the body.

+ Press the outer rim of your palms into the floor.

+ Spread your fingers.

+ Slightly dome up through the centre of your hand as if you were hiding a delicate flower. Traction your fingers.

+ Engage your forearms by turning two imaginary dials—the right hand turns isometrically to the right, and the left to the left. Your hands don't move.

BREATHE

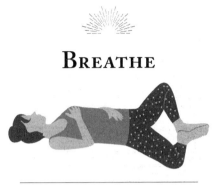

TUNE INTO THE BREATH

Sometimes it seems so difficult to take just one more breath.
I want to teach you how to breathe again as an act of self-care.
It will be beautiful.

To the Mind

Pra: bring forth; to breathe

Prana: the life force that animates all existence, or that which causes animation of life force

Ayama: to stretch or expand life force

Pranayama: breathing in and breathing out with conscious awareness to encourage balance and harmony of internal energy

Themes: the breath, subtle body, energy, creating awareness, mindfulness

LANGUAGE OF THE BREATH

Be breathed
Breathe freely
Siphon the air
Follow the breath
Treasure your breath
Fluid, beautiful breath
Homogenise the breath
Express the inhale fully
Let yourself be breathed
Let the breath move you

Call the breath back home
Breathe to create openings
Dedicate every breath to x
Exhale and let go of gravity
Let the exhale take the pose
Breathe into your back body
Turn your breath into patience
Follow the source of the breath
Find alignment with your breath
Move in the current of your breath

Even out the texture of your breath

Every inhale is an opportunity for x

Layer the practice breath by breath

Look at the breath at a cellular level

Feel the soft cloth of your diaphragm

Zoom in on the quality of your breath

Pour consciousness into your breathing

Let the breath move you to new depths

Feel the oceanic fullness in each breath

Feel the breath sink like water into sand

Weave the breath in and out of the poses

Let each exhalation carry a wave of release

Sweep the breath through your body house

Find a patient steady quality in your breath

Feel your ribs open and close like fish gills

Breathe like a baby; feel the belly rise and fall

Allow your breath to move from the inside out

Let your mind find a resting place in the breath

Let the breath expand through your inner territory

Feel the breath move in your body like tidal gravity

Invite the breath to become slower, deeper, smoother

Let the breath lead you in and through the movements

Use your breath to determine the pace of your practice

Breathe as if you were soaking your lungs in a fine mist

Follow your breath to the place where effortlessness arises

Exhale as if you were pouring olive oil in a long thin stream

Offer your exhale to the past and your inhale to your present

Feel the colour of your breath spread like ink into blotting paper

Feel the tentacles of the breath spread to every seam in the body

Let the breath be the resonating factor that motivates your practice

The inhale and exhale are skirts of a jellyfish, moving up and down

Use your breath to harness the power that lives in the present moment

When you breathe imagine you are opening and closing venetian blinds

The inhale slowly takes you from the dark of the ocean to the clear blue surface

As you inhale the universe inhales into you, as you exhale you breathe into the universe

To the Heart

Eastern medicine believes *prana*, or *qi*, is the animating force of our life. It permeates us down to a cellular level and is responsible for the way things move within us. The way qi moves or doesn't move in the organs and *meridians* (pathways) directly affects our mental, physical, and emotional health. When we bring awareness to how we breathe, we have the capacity to align ourselves with health.

> *Ancient yogis believed we are blessed with so many breaths for our life.*
> *If this is so, why not stretch our life out a bit longer by taking slow breaths?*
> *We begin our life on an inhale and end it on an exhale.*
> *The part in between is our dance with life.*
> *Make it a beautiful dance.*

Every day we rise and breathe up to 23,000 times into our lives, our dramas, our fears, and our days, without much thought. Breathing is the only autonomous system of the body that we can also control. This means that the body governs it, but like a magnet moving metal shavings, we have the ability to consciously use our breath to focus and move prana through the body-mind.

Our breath and mind are closely linked. When we concentrate on breathing practices, we tether the wild horse of the mind, which produces a relaxed awareness. Like two sides of the same coin, how we breathe is an indicator of our mood and our mood is an indicator of our breath. Changing how we breathe is one of the quickest ways to alter our mood.

If we use breath awareness in our poses, we get to explore how far or deep we should go and when we need to yield and surrender. If we move with the breath, we become sensitive to the ever-changing needs of the body. Without awareness we are less likely to discover the places in the pose we have vacated, or we are more likely to override strong sensations, which may lead to injury.

> *The breath flows in and just before it turns to flow out,*
> *There is a flash of pure joy, life is renewed.*
> *Awaken into that.*
> *The Radiance Sutras*
>
> Lorin Roche

To the Body

❧ *Tune into the Breath* ☙

DIAPHRAGM WRAP

1. In a seated position, wrap a strap around your diaphragm, not too tight or too loose.

2. Hold the strap in your hands.

3. As you inhale, feel your ribs expand three-dimensionally, contracting the strap and pulling it a little tighter.

4. As you breathe out, feel the strap slowly loosen its grip.

LUNG CRADLE

1. Lie down on the floor.

2. Cross your right hand over your ribs and cradle your left lung in your hand as if you were holding it.

3. Breathe into your right hand and see if you can feel the side of your lung inflate, the front of your lung and the back of your lung.

4. Repeat on the other side.

ROLLING BRIDGE

This helps students to understand tempo and acclimates them to taking full inhales and exhales to completion.

1. Start in Bridge pose with your arms by your side.

2. As you breathe in, lift your hands over your head to touch the floor behind you.

3. As you breathe out, bring your hands back down by your sides. Your hands should touch the floor at the tip of the inhale and the end of the exhale.

COBRA ROLL

This helps students attune to lengthening the exhale while in the poses.

1. Lie on your belly and place your hands on the floor near your shoulders.

2. Inhale for a count of four; lift your chest.

3. Exhale for a count of six or eight as you lower your chest back down.

Visualisation: The cobra listens through its belly, feeling the vibrations of the earth into its being.

SIDE BODY BREATH

1. Bend your knees and place your feet wide on the edges of the mat. Drop your knees to the right.

2. Stretch your arms up over your head and bind your left wrist with your right hand.

3. Pull your left wrist gently.

4. This exposes more of your left lung.

5. Breathe into your left lung.

6. Repeat on the other side.

BACK BODY BREATH

1. Place the block under your thoracic spine, around where the tips of your shoulder blades lie.

2. Breathe into the back of your body where the block meets your ribs.

CACTUS BREATH FLOW

1. Sit comfortably.

2. Open your arms out at shoulder height and bend your elbows to form 'cactus' arms.

3. Inhale and feel the expanse across your chest.

4. Exhale, bring your inner forearms to touch and your open palms to face you. Repeat several times.

5. Finish with your hands in Anjali mudra/ namaste.

························ *Tune into the Breath* ························

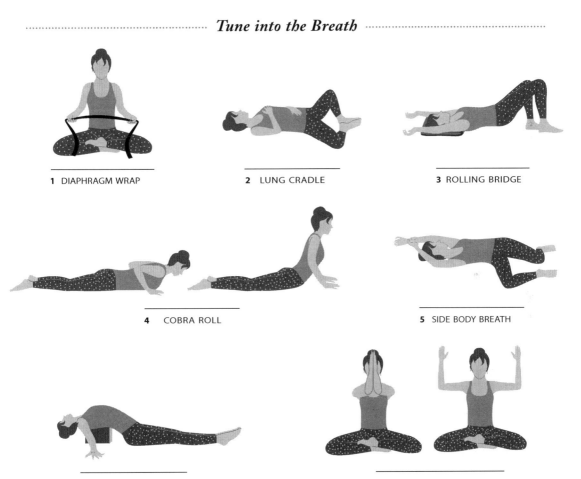

1 DIAPHRAGM WRAP

2 LUNG CRADLE

3 ROLLING BRIDGE

4 COBRA ROLL

5 SIDE BODY BREATH

6 BACK BODY BREATH

7 CACTUS BREATH FLOW

Teaching Notes

+ Imagine your lungs are like Venetian blinds. On each inhale the blinds blink open and on each exhale they close.

+ The space between each breath is the bridge between our inner and outer worlds. Let the relationship be harmonious.

+ Imagine your breath filling you three-dimensionally: to the side of your ribs, the front and back of your body, up to your throat, and down to your pelvic floor.

+ At the end of the exhale feel a slight contraction at the base of your pelvic floor. At the end of the inhale feel the pelvic floor relax and spread.

+ Sense the breath delicately opening and closing your nostrils like the wings of a butterfly.

Pranayama is the fourth limb of yoga after yama, niyama, and asana. This gives you a clue as to how the ancient yogis viewed what needs to happen before we begin breathing exercises. In the modern day setting and with time restraints, consider introducing the following three elements before pranayama.

+ Relaxing the nervous system through Savasana or through a restorative pose or poses.

+ Opening the side of the body with side stretches such as lying Banana pose.

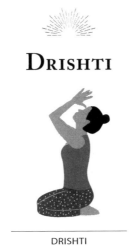

DRISHTI

DRISHTI

People are not disturbed by things, but by the views they take of them.
EPICTETUS

To the Mind

Drishti: to hold one's attention internally or on a point of focus and in doing so, steady the movements of the mind. Our way of viewing the world.

Themes: insight, attention and focus, world view, sensory withdrawal

LANGUAGE OF SIGHT

Relax the muscles around the eyes
Let the skin around the eyes soften
Let your two eyes become one soft eye
Make your eyes wide like Buddha eyes
Close down the curtains of your eyes
Let your eyes deepen in their sockets
Release the lines of tension between the eyes
See the whole picture, have a bird's eye view of life
Where do you go when you close your eyes, what do you see?

To the Heart

Drishti has many meanings. In Ayurveda it is the centre of the retina, in ashtanga yoga it is referred to as focussed attention, and in Mahayana Buddhism drishti is the practice of constantly challenging our world view. Drishti is the precursor to *pratyahara*, or sensory withdrawal, the practice of drawing your attention inwards to move you into a state of meditation.

Drishti practices allow us to look without judging, see without attaching, focus without hardness.

When we dart our eyes, close our lids, wander off in the mind, or form a story about what we see, we are practicing the opposite of drishti.

Our brain uses fifty percent of its functioning capacity just to process what we see.[3] Drishti is the practice of fine tuning our vision and processing what we see through a clearer lens.

Ya drishti, sa srishti
How we view the world affects our reality

The skill of really 'seeing' is highlighted in the Japanese art of *kintsugi*. Artists mend broken bowls with slivers of gold to highlight the imperfections. This love of seeing things anew for the first time is a reminder that beauty is everywhere if we know how to look. When we look at something, we pass it through the filters of what we know—our conditioning, perceptions, and stories. We see things, as Anais Nin said, 'as we are' rather than as they are. This filtered binocular vision is illustrated in the Vedic parable, *The Rope and the Snake*.

THE ROPE AND THE SNAKE

A man is walking along a forest path at dusk. In the dim of the light, he sees a poisonous snake and in terror he turns and runs back the way he came.

The next day, as he returns along the same path, he finds a coiled rope on the ground. He realises that in the darkness, he mistook the coiled rope as a snake and it dawns on him that in the dark it is hard to see reality as it truly is, but in the light of day, we see more clearly.

---

[3] "MIT Research—Brain Processing of Visual Information," MIT News, Massachusetts Institute of Technology, 1996. http://news.mit.edu/1996/visualprocessing

To the Body

❧ *Drishti* ☙

GLABELLA MASSAGE

Acupressure applied to the third eye centre between the eyebrows is said to help you sleep better, calm anxiety, and relieve tension headaches. It also helps quieten the brain, soothe the muscles of the eyes, and helps the body relax as a whole.

1. Come into Child's pose.
2. Place a block under your brow and a soft towel on the block.
3. Massage the point between your eyebrows by rocking your forehead side-to-side slowly.
4. Feel release around the muscles of your eyes, especially between your eyes.

LION'S BREATH

1. From Child's pose, lift your torso so you are sitting on your calves upright.
2. Close your eyes, inhale through your nostrils.
3. Open your eyes, exhale through your mouth. As you exhale, stick your tongue out and look up towards the spot between your eyes.

PALMING

1. Come into Seated Wide Leg or Straddle pose.
2. Place a block between your legs.
3. Place your elbows on your legs.
4. Turn your palms up and rest your eye sockets in the palms of your hands.

TRATAKA (FIXED GAZE MEDITATION)

1. Light a candle and place it on the floor in front of you.
2. Sit in a comfortable Easy Seat posture.
3. Stare into the flame with soft eyes. The eyes will begin to water and self-clean.

DRISHTI MEDITATION

Bring your attention to the point between the eyes; soften here, let it spread.

Relax the muscles around your eyes, let them deepen and retract from the job of looking. as they deepen into their sockets, retracting from the job of looking.

Under your lids make your eyes wide and soft like Buddha eyes, as if you can see everything in perspective.

As your gaze softens, your mind quietens and your energy is preserved.

Drishti is the art of seeing things as they are, rather than how we think they are; it is the sight within the sight.

See the patterns of light play out under your lids, watch them move and morph.

Bring your attention up and to the point between your eyes.

Stay here for a few moments.

When you are ready to return, rub your hands, place them over your eyes, and blink your eyes open.

Slowly remove your hands and get ready to move and flow.

Drishti

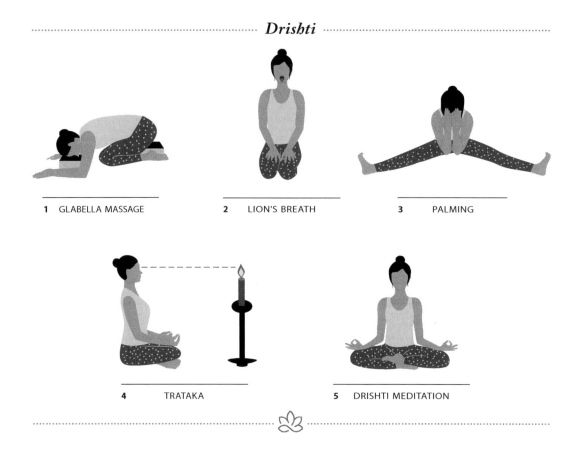

| **1** GLABELLA MASSAGE | **2** LION'S BREATH | **3** PALMING |

| **4** TRATAKA | **5** DRISHTI MEDITATION |

Teaching Notes

+ To round the theme into a complete class, incorporate drishti focus points from the ashtanga tradition. Focus students' attention on the tips of their noses, thumbs, third eyes, etc.

+ Eye yoga can be done to strengthen the muscles of the eyes. Look up to the right upper corner of your eyes, left lower corner, straight up and straight down. This can be done with the eyes open or closed.

+ Focussing on something in the distance will relieve eye strain.

+ In Eagle pose, encourage soft vision and a steady gaze as if you were an eagle homing in on a target.

+ A drishti theme complements sixth chakra work.

+ Candle-gazing practice encourages softening of the seeing eyes, cleanses the eyes, and is a good practice to do prior to meditation.

STHIRA MEETS SUKHA

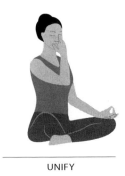

UNIFY

The soft overcomes the hard.
LAO TZU

To the Mind

Sukha: softness, ease, calm, comfort, tranquil, contented, restful, humble, good space.

An older translation of sukha referred to the relationship of the axle to a wheel. The axle needs to be the right length for the wheel to turn smoothly.

Sthira: strong, steady, grounded, firmly rooted, held in place, present, resolute, steadfast, dynamic

Asanam: seat

Sthira sukham asanam: The seat is steady and comfortable. Equipoise arises when the two qualities of effort and ease are balanced both in the body and the mind.

Themes: balance, ease, equanimity, duality

LANGUAGE OF STHIRA AND SUKHA

Effort and ease

Push and yield

Sun and moon

Yang and yin

Dark and light

Push and pull
Matter and spirit
Effort and surrender
Giving and receiving
Balance and imbalance
Flexible and inflexible
Strength and flexibility
Tension and relaxation
Awareness and sensitivity
Strengths and limitations
Holding on and letting go
Engagement and letting go
Drawing in and expanding out

To the Heart

Patanjali tells us that if we can find the sweet spot within effort, we will have entered the state of asana, which is balanced, easeful, and takes the path of least resistance. T.K.V. Desikachar says that to find this ease and balance, we must attain relaxation without dullness and alertness without tension. The closer we are to ease, the further our distance from dis-ease.

Life veers between two opposing forces. Like yin and yang, to find equilibrium, we must continually work with this constant push and pull to find an even keel. Too much sukha and we stagnate, too much sthira and we deplete.

To the Body

❧ *Unify* ☙

Sama: equal, same

Vritti: fluctuations, movement, disturbance

Sama Vritti Breathing: an equal ratio breath where the inhales and exhales are balanced. (Square Breathing is where the inhales, exhales, and retentions are the same ratio.)

Take your seat.

Feel into your spine. Teeter back and forth to find equipoise in your posture.

Find sthira in your spine, alertness but softness, signalling you are ready to practice.

Pranayama is a process to find comfort within the discomfort and balance within the imbalances.

Conscious breathing soothes and helps us find peace in what is being presented, balancing effort and ease.

SINGLE NOSTRIL BREATHING

Known as Single or Alternate Nostril Breathing, *Nadi Shodhana, Anuloma Viloma*

This technique balances the left and the right hemispheres of the brain, the sthira and sukha sides. By playing with variations of this practice, we create unity in our mind and step out of duality, right and wrong, you and me, them and us. When we stabilise our mind this way, the chatter of the divided mind subsides.

When we are soaked in calmness, we can make confident choices, step away from confusion, and see our vision or path with clarity.

Yogis believe that our energy is regulated by three channels, or rivers, called *nadis*. On the left is *ida*, and on the right *pingala*. By manipulating the prana in the causeways of our breath, we can alter our states of being and balance the central channel, or *sushumna*.

Science has shown that during the day, we switch between breathing predominantly in the right and left nostrils. Alternating dominance has been attributed to swelling of the tissues in either the right or left sides, slowing the breath. It is estimated this sway between right and left nostrils switches every two to eight hours, juggling our energy between energetic and restful states, sympathetic activity and parasympathetic activity.[4]

When we balance the polarities between sthira and sukha, *rajas* (energetic, active, dynamic) and *tamas* (dullness, inertia, inactivity), we enter the state of yoga.

ALTERNATE NOSTRIL BREATHING

When we inhale, we stimulate energy; when we exhale, we calm energy. Imagine the breath as fine silk or a scent you love. Find smoothness in the texture of the breath.

---

[4] Dhandayutham Ashwini, "Effect of Left & Right Nostril Breathing on R-R Interval Among Adult Males—A Cross-Sectional Study," *International Journal of Biomedical Research* 06, no. 2 (February 2015): 87-91. https://ssjournals.com/index.php/ijbr/issue/view/208

1. Sit at ease.
2. Block off your right nostril with your right thumb.
3. Inhale through your left nostril.
4. Block off your left nostril with your right ring finger.

5. Exhale through your right nostril.
6. Inhale through your right nostril.

Repeat this pattern for ten cycles.

VARIATIONS ON ALTERNATE NOSTRIL BREATHING

SUKHA: MOON SHOWER

When we inhale through the left nostril, we stimulate the ida nerve ending. Ida is the feminine, relaxing, calming, receptive, lunar, tamas, or sukha side.

1. Place your left hand on your lap in Gyan mudra with your thumb and first finger connected. Your palm is turned up and your three fingers slightly curled.
2. Block off your right nostril with your right thumb.
3. Inhale through your left nostril and out of your left nostril.

STHIRA: SUN SHOWER

When we inhale through the right nostril, we stimulate the pingala nerve ending. Pingala is the masculine, yang, solar, rajasic, or sthira side.

1. Place your right hand on your lap in Gyan mudra with your thumb and first finger connected. Your palm is turned up, and your three fingers slightly curled.
2. Block off your left nostril with your left ring finger.
3. Inhale through your right nostril and out of your right nostril.

STHIRA WITH SHARP EXHALES

1. Block off your left nostril with your ring finger.
2. Inhale through your right nostril.
3. Hold the breath at its apex for a beat.
4. Exhale 80 percent sharply through your right nostril.
5. Finish the exhale with a smooth breath right to the end.
6. Repeat for ten rounds.

For Sukha with Sharp Exhales, repeat this exercise, breathing in through your left side with short forceful exhales through your left nostril.

STHIRA AND SUKHA EXHALES

1. Inhale through both nostrils.
2. Block off your right nostril with your thumb.
3. Breath out through your left nostril.
4. Release your thumb.
5. Inhale through both nostrils.
6. Block off your left nostril with your ring finger.
7. Exhale through your right nostril.

VISUAL STHIRA AND SUKHA

This practice uses the power of visualisation to breathe in and out through the nostrils.

It's a soothing precursor to Savasana.

1. Lie down in Savasana.
2. Inhale a long slow, smooth breath through both nostrils.
3. Exhale through both nostrils.
4. Visualise your right nostril.
5. Without using your fingers, imagine blocking off your right nostril and breathing a long slow breath through the left nostril.
6. Exhale through your left nostril.
7. Inhale through your left nostril.
8. Imagine blocking off your left nostril in your mind's eye and slowly exhale through your right nostril.
9. Repeat steps 1 to 6 for ten rounds.

Teaching Notes

+ Squeezing and lifting out of poses and setting strong foundations while engaging muscles will bring in sthira. Flexible students will benefit from this approach.

+ Is your natural tendency to overdo or push too hard? How would it feel to not go so deep in the poses? Use blocks to create a visual reminder to back out of poses. Take two steps back from the edge of the cliff.

+ Is your natural tendency to take things easy, back off when things get difficult and give up? Understand these inclinations and vote to stay or put in more effort. Kundalini practices shine a light on your relationship to staying power with vigorous poses lasting up to three minutes.

+ If you want more sthira in your life, challenge your mindset with a faster-flowing salutation or a more extended hold in poses. Consider experimenting with a posture you would rather avoid.

+ Does your mind wander during the poses or Savasana? Do your eyes dart? Zoning out indicates loss of sthira.

+ Use an anchor such as your breath to cultivate the steadiness of the mind. If you lose your breath's silkiness during the postures, it is an indication you are moving away from sukha. Back off or rest until you find the steady tempo again.

+ Monitor which nostril's breath is more dominant in Single Nostril Breathing and adapt your practice to balance that energy. Right nostril domination is active energy and left nostril domination is passive energy.

+ Invite and play with opposites in your practice so you can reside in equanimity.

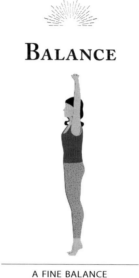

BALANCE

A FINE BALANCE

Choose rather to be strong of soul than strong of body.
Pythagoras

To the Mind

Tula/tola: balance

Many yoga poses require us to find balance. In the process of doing so we learn to find our centre, the unmoving place within that is not affected by turbulence without. Balance requires us to find equilibrium with gravity and when we find it, we also find stillness within the body and mind.

Themes: balance, support, equanimity, resilience

LANGUAGE OF BALANCE

Nature strives for balance

Find equilibrium/equipoise

Equanimity, equal standing

Balance like a see-saw/carpenter's level/scales

Balance front to back, top to bottom, side to side

Like a tug of war, find the balance between push and pull/holding on and letting go

Balance is the act of assessing where you are and adjusting yourself to come back to centre

To the Heart

Consider resilience in action. Why does one building collapse and another stand tall during times of shift and turbulence? Why does one person fall and another bounce back from adversity?

Balance practices embody the key elements of resilience:
- To stay present and anchored.
- To be able to adapt to your environment.
- To have the resources to rise up after you fall.

Resilience
When life is literally in free fall,
when all our support systems have been snatched away,
remember that you can only fall as far as the ground
and the ground is love itself.
From here, you will harness your inner resources,
or someone will help you up,
and you will be ready to start again.
You may have stumbled; the path may have crumbled,
but you are still on the course.

To the Body

ꙮ *A Fine Balance* ꙮ

PENDULUM
1. Stand on both feet with your left arm straight up to the sky.
2. Put your weight into your left leg. Put your right hand on your hip.
3. Inhale, swing your left arm away from your head about thirty degrees and your right leg out to the side at about thirty degrees.
4. Exhale, bring your arm and foot back to the midline.
5. Repeat five to ten times.
6. Repeat on the other side.

TIP TOE BALANCE

1. Stand with your feet slightly wider than hip-width apart.

2. Interlace your hands above your head with your palms turned upwards.

3. As you inhale, lift onto your toes and stretch your hands to the ceiling.

4. Exhale, lower your heels.

5. Repeat four to five times.

HIGH HEELED CHAIR

1. Come into Chair with your knees bent and your arms overhead.

2. Inhale, lift on to your toes with your knees bent.

3. Exhale, drop your heels down and your arms by your sides.

4. Repeat four to five times.

BLOCK TREE

1. Stand with your left foot on a block. If you need support, turn side-on and place your left hand on a wall.

2. Swing your right leg back and forth freely four or five times.

3. On the last swing, bring your knee up to your chest and hook it with your right hand.

4. Stay and balance here.

5. Place your right foot onto your thigh or calf and balance in Block Tree for five long slow breaths.

6. Repeat on the other side.

MOUNTAIN

1. Stand in Mountain.

2. Close your eyes.

3. Gently sway side-to-side, feeling the moving, shifting weight beneath you.

4. Come to the middle and stand there, equanimous.

5. Sense into the ripples of movement that keep you upright.

A fine Balance

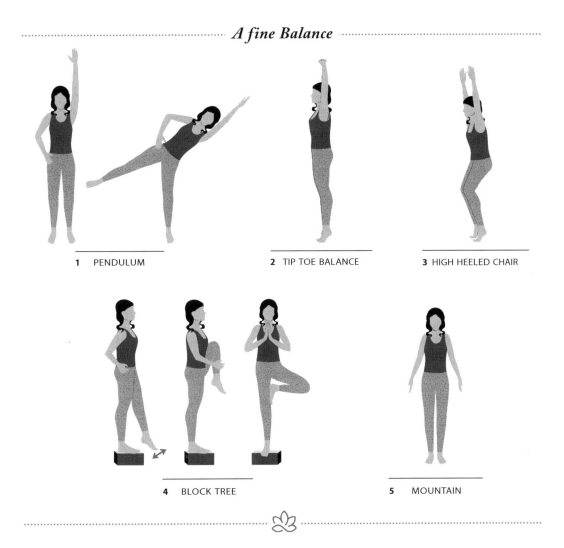

| 1 PENDULUM | 2 TIP TOE BALANCE | 3 HIGH HEELED CHAIR |

| 4 BLOCK TREE | 5 MOUNTAIN |

Teaching Notes

✦ Balancing poses force us to find a confluence of compression and tension in our body. To balance on one leg or our arms is to dive into our centre of gravity, to be grounded, and to develop resiliency.

✦ When we balance, if we fix our ankle steadfastly and someone pushes us, we will topple like a brick building. Instead imagine that your feet are stabilisers, taking and absorbing the movements and attenuating them through your body.

+ When we stand on one foot the tendency is for the ankle to roll out on the standing foot. Encourage more pressure onto the medial line of the standing foot.

+ Encourage use of a wall to find support in any balance posture.

+ Note that in balance postures the foundation moves to accommodate the balance. Remind students balance isn't about force or strength but moving to meet the changing nature of what is being presented.

+ One of the goals of yoga and a healthy life is to come back into balance. We can only do this when we know we are out of balance.

+ See Mountain pose for more ideas on balance.

SPINAL RIVER

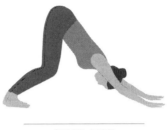

SPINAL RIVER

There is the mud, and there is the lotus that grows out of the mud.
We need the mud in order to make the lotus.

THICH NHAT HANH

To the Mind

NEUTRAL SPINE

When the spine is neutral, the four curves of the spine are present:

- the outwards curve of the sacrum
- the inwards curve of the lumbar
- the outwards curve of the thoracic
- the inwards curve of the cervical

THE MOVEMENTS OF THE SPINE

The spine has six movements:

- twisting left
- twisting right
- forward folding
- back bending
- side bending left
- side bending right

AXIAL EXTENSION

In addition to these movements, the spine moves in an 'upwards,' lengthening movement along its axis. This helps create decompression and space between each individual vertebra, counters the effects of gravity, and brings awareness to posture. It can be experienced in Mountain, Downward Facing Dog, Plank, Handstand, Headstand, and poses where we 'stretch' the arms away from the legs to lengthen the spine and temporarily 'flatten' the curves of the spine rather like the spine of a book.

Themes: subtle energy, foundational poses, chakra system

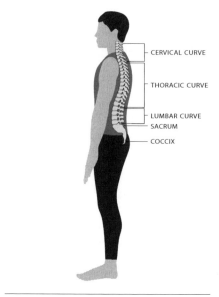

CERVICAL CURVE

THORACIC CURVE

LUMBAR CURVE
SACRUM

COCCIX

THE FOUR CURVES OF THE SPINE

LANGUAGE OF THE SPINE

Serpentine spine

Your stegosaurus spine

The swing bridge of bones

Extend your spine like an antenna

Feel the imprint of your spine into the mat

Lay your spine down like a string of precious beads

Imagine your spine coiling and turning like a helix around its axis

Feel the spine rise up from its base like a snake peering up and over its basket

As you twist, feel as if you were walking up the spiral staircase of your spine

Imagine your spine like seaweed, buoyant and flexible, moving with the waters of your body

To the Heart

The spiritual spine stands sentinel, holding the shape of our bones and the clay of our muscles to attention in life.

The giver and receiver of messages, this serpentine river is the channeler of energy both masculine and feminine. In Tantra it is said that at the base of the spine, a serpent waits ready to rise up.

This axial highway of bones is responsible for maintaining posture, protecting the message centre of our spinal cord, and enabling movement.

Like the stem of a lotus or the trunk of a tree, the atlas bone supports our skull and brain. This topmost cervical bone is appropriately named after the Greek deity Atlas, who holds the weight of the world on his shoulders for eternity.

To the Body

❧ *The River of Life* ☙

Yogis have long maintained that you can tell the health and longevity of a person by the health of their spine.

This simple warm-up practice takes the spine through its range of movements and brings attention to our centre line. It then plays with some 'traction' postures to imitate spinal decompression.

SPINAL STIR

1. Sit in Easy Seat posture.
2. Start to circle your spine in a circular action for at least a minute. Imagine you are stirring the pile of bones in one continuous movement.
3. Repeat in an anticlockwise direction.

LOW BACK SEATED CAT-COW

1. Place your hands on your shins.
2. Move the base of your spine (lumbar) forwards and back in a Cat-Cow movement.
3. Continue this movement for at least one minute, gathering speed towards the end.
4. Try to isolate the movement in your low back.

UPPER BACK SEATED CAT-COW

1. Take your attention to your mid-back (thoracic) spine.
2. Open your arms out to the sides.
3. Inhale, arch your back, and turn your palms up.
4. Exhale, rotate your arms down, and flex your back.
5. Continue for one minute.

SEATED TWIST

1. Change the cross of your legs.
2. Use your core to turn your torso to the right.
3. Place your left hand on your right knee and your right hand on the floor behind you for support.
4. Repeat on the other side.

LATERAL CHILD

1. Come into Child's pose.
2. Stretch your arms out and your seat back towards your heels.
3. Stay here for a few breaths.
4. Walk your torso to the right.

5. Stay here and breathe into your left side.
6. Repeat on the other side.

DANGLING

1. Lift your hips up and walk your hands back to your feet.
2. Bend at your knees and traction your spine over your legs.
3. Hold your elbows.
4. Let the weight of your head drop.

TRACTION DOWN DOG

1. Find a partner.
2. Place a strap around your partner's upper thighs.
3. Take the ends of the strap in both hands.
4. Take a wide stance or stagger your legs. Bend your legs.
5. Lean back and pull up and out on the strap.
6. Put as much weight as you need to into the strap so your partner's hands become light and hover off the floor.

The river of Life

1 SPINAL STIR

2 LOW BACK
CAT COW

3 UPPER BACK
CAT COW

4 SEATED TWIST

5 LATERAL CHILD

6 DANGLING

7 TRACTION
DOWN DOG

Teaching Notes

✦ Aim to take students through all movements of the spine in a class.

✦ Remember to cue vertebra as singular. *Roll up out of the posture one vertebra at a time, or find space between each veterbra. Conversely, lengthen the entire veterbrae.*

MEDITATION—SPIRITUAL CAIRNS

Sit in a posture that allows you to feel at ease.

Take your attention to your internal landscape.

Feel the stack of spinal bones, tail, low back, mid back, and neck.

Feel the four curves of your spine, like a wave, present and stable.

A cairn is a stack of stones, one on top of the other forming a tower or balance.

To place one stone on top of another like a spinal column requires patience and presence.

Each rock carries its own grace and spirit and can be placed as a spiritual practice, to offer thanks or as a prayer for someone in need. Built across time and cultures, they can be a marker for someone who is lost on their journey, a memorial for the deceased, or a symbolic abode to meditate on.

One on top of the other, the stones form a spine which is grounded, centred, and aligned. Each stone, each bone, represents and supports the one above and below, a natural reminder of union and connection.

As you get ready to practice, name your bones, or stones. Who or what would you like to send your prayer, thanks, or guidance to today?

MEDITATION—BACK BODY SUPPORT

The yogis say the back of the body is where we hold on to life and the front is where we project into life. By relaxing the back of the body, we truly learn to let go.

Lie down on your mat and take a moment to get comfortable. Let your pelvis be heavy. Feel the four curves of your back, the sacred bone, the lumbar, the dorsal spine, and the back of the throat start to release to the floor. Let the weight of the world drop.

Soften and snuggle your shoulders back and down and feel a release, as if you were taking off a heavy backpack.

Now take a long slow breath down the length of your spine and feel as if you are feeding the entire information highway, the stack of bones that holds you upright from day to day.

The spine represents your support system. And through its intelligence it will inform you of where you need to pay attention, or where you need to let go. If you are not supported in any way, your body will not lie to you.

Take your attention to your upper back, neck, and shoulders. Relax the large guy ropes on the side of the neck and the muscles on the side of your throat. This area represents what we 'shoulder' or take on upon ourselves, the self-imposed pressures, the demands we make.

Relax here. Take off your backpack. Set yourself free.

Take your attention to your mid back. This area represents relationships, community. Here we may harbour obligations from the outside world, as if the world is pressuring us to perform and live up to others' expectations.

Relax here. Take off your backpack. Set yourself free.

Take your attention to the soft curve in your low back. This is your connection to ancestry and represents the support we were given as infants.

If it feels right for you, bring to mind a part of your life where you need some support right now. Maybe it's a project you need to complete or some difficulty you are working through. If this is not you at the moment, then call to mind someone who needs your support. Picture the situation and try to get a sense of where you feel this in your back body.

Now let go of the story and sit with the feeling in your back. Watch it move and resonate.

When you are ready, softly blink open your eyes, roll onto one side into foetal position before you get ready to go out into your life.

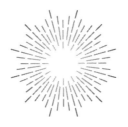

CHAPTER FIVE

STARTING SHAPES

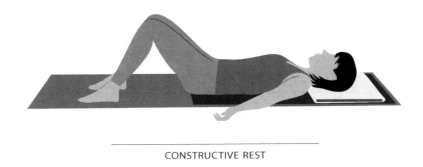

CONSTRUCTIVE REST

Be still, stillness reveals the secrets of eternity

Lao Tzu

By getting grounded early on and entering into a relationship with our bodies, we become a physical conduit for the teachings. This section focuses on getting you out of your head and into your body by bringing attention to the most loved starting poses, their variations, and words to soothe.

When we take on the shape of any pose, we embody the teachings behind it. We become the earth, the tree, the child, and they in part become us.

WHY PRACTICE?

In the stillness of the morning, in the early quietness of your breath, the practice is preparing you.

The strength you need for the Warriors won't let you fall when your world crumbles.

The solidarity of Mountain pose will make you stand tall and remind you to follow your dreams when others doubt you.

The balance poses will bring you back to centre when you are caught off guard.

The intensity of long holds will remind you to not give up.

Every transition you make with grace will shore you up for the unexpected twists and turns of your life.

Your band of resilience will expand to encompass all of life's comings and goings with every pose you want to leave—but stay in.

And all the people around you, that practice with you, have shown up to remind you that you are not alone in this.

All of this work has led you to where you are now.

It is making you exemplary and giving you clarity.

Slowly but surely, it melts your vagueness and fears, unleashing your goodness, creativity, and love.

Easy Seat

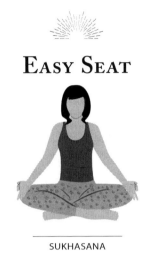

SUKHASANA

Until you make the unconscious conscious,
it will direct your life and you will call it fate.
CARL JUNG

To the Mind

Sukha: ease, happiness, joy, bliss that is a lasting state

Sukhasana: Easy Seat pose, often used for meditation

Themes: santosha or contentment, finding ease, happiness, meditation

BENEFITS

+ creates flexibility in the knee and hip joints
+ requires strength to hold and support the trunk, strengthening the back
+ grounding, calming pose
+ taps into the energy of the root chakra

To the Heart

Also known as Burmese posture, Easy Seat pose is not as simple as it looks. The hips need to be open and the back strong and alert, which can be difficult for those not accustomed to sitting on floors. Historically, yogis practiced poses solely for the benefit of their meditation practice, so they could sit comfortably for long periods of time. In Sukhasana, when the spine is aligned and arises from a stable base, the experience of meditation changes from one of fighting with our body to one of non-judgemental awareness.

This makes Sukhasana the perfect pose for investigating what we have brought to our practice with us physically and mentally.

To the Body

❧ Seated Warm-ups ❧

SETTING UP FOR SUKHASANA

Sit comfortably, and cross your legs. If you need to support your seat, knees, or ankles with blocks or blankets, use those now to hold you in ease.

Be at ease here.

Take your attention to your tail, your root. In your mind's eye, draw the energy of the tail bone towards the pubic bone.

Take your attention to your sit bones. Like two heels, feel them balanced evenly on the ground left and right, and gently squeeze them towards one another.

From this diamond of support—the two sit bones, the pubic bone, and the tailbone—feel a lift up into the base of your spine.

Follow this lift up through your back, into your neck and head. Align yourself over this centre line.

Bring your thumbs to your armpits, lift the skin up and spread it back, and now relax your arms by your sides.

Untangle any knots in your jaw.

Let your outer shape be a reflection of your inner self.

Now take your attention to your spine, the conduit of your life.

As you breathe in, pull the breath up from the tail, the root, right up to the atlas bone that holds your head.

Exhale, release your breath down your spine.

Keep going like this, creating awareness.

Awareness is a light you shine in and on yourself.

Feel yourself light up like a lighthouse, spreading the awareness in all directions.

Sit comfortably in Sukhasana or one of her variations.

CACTUS FLOWER

1. Inhale, bring your elbows to shoulder height with the arms in a cactus shape. Lift up and arch your upper back.
2. Exhale, flex your back, bring the forearms together and tuck the head down.

CACTUS CORE

1. Inhale, bring your elbows to shoulder height with your arms in a cactus shape.
2. Short sharp exhale; turn to the right from your core.
3. Come back to centre.
4. Short sharp exhale; turn again to the right.
5. The inhale will come naturally as you return to the centre.
6. The exhale is through your nostrils.
7. Repeat to the left.

EAGLE ARMS

1. Wrap your right arm under your left.
2. Lift your elbows.
3. Take your hands away from your face.
4. Repeat on the other side.

HUGGING CIRCLES

1. Cross your arms over your chest and hold your shoulders.
2. Make circular movements from your upper body in a clockwise then anticlockwise pattern.

OPEN AND CLOSE TO SEATED TWIST

1. Twist to your right.
2. Bring your right hand behind your ear.
3. Inhale, open your right elbow out to the right.
4. Exhale, curl your right elbow towards your left knee.
5. Repeat the open and close movement five times.
6. After the last 'open,' place your right hand behind you on the floor and twist to your right.
7. Repeat on the left side.

SEATED FORWARD FOLD

1. Inhale, lengthen up through the front of the body.
2. Exhale, bow forwards, and place your hands on the floor or on blocks.
3. Squeeze your sit bones together.

Seated Warm-ups

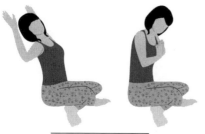

1 CACTUS FLOWER

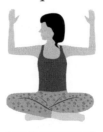

2 CACTUS CORE

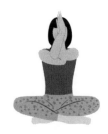

3 EAGLE ARMS

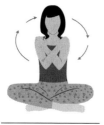

4 HUGGING CIRCLES

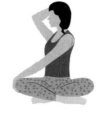

5 OPEN AND CLOSE

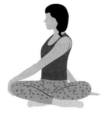

6 SEATED TWIST

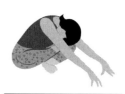

7 SEATED FORWARD FOLD

Lotus Variations

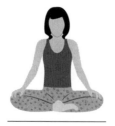

1 BIDDHASANA

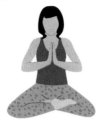

2 QUARTER LOTUS

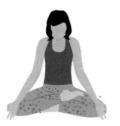

3 HALF LOTUS

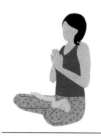

4 FULL LOTUS

Teaching Notes

Below are some seated posture variations.

❧ *Siddhasana* ☙

Siddha: accomplished
In this variation both heels are pulled into the groin. Both feet remain on the floor.

❧ *Lotus (Padma) variations* ☙

QUARTER LOTUS	HALF LOTUS	FULL LOTUS
Bend your right knee and move your right foot on the floor in front of your left sit bone. Place your left foot on top of the right inner shin.	Bring your right foot into your groin. Place your left ankle on top of your right thigh close to the groin.	Bring your right foot on top of your left leg close to your groin. Place your left foot on top of your right thigh close to the groin.

KNEES TO CHEST

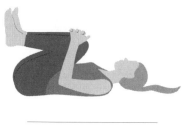

KNEES TO CHEST

The practice of yoga brings us face to face
with the extraordinary complexity of our own being.
SRI AUROBINDO

To the Mind

Apana: downwards-moving life force

Asana: seat

Apanasana: Knees to Chest pose

Themes: digestion, detox, air element, potential, vata (air and space) balancing

BENEFITS

+ helps expel and move internal winds

+ massages the internal organs, especially in the low body

+ firmly compresses the lower body, aiding circulation

+ stretches the low back

+ lifting the head to the knees strengthens the back and abdominal muscles

+ rocking from side-to-side irons out the creases in the low back

To the Heart

In yoga the word for seed is *bija*. Bija is the beginning or where everything in nature originated.

We all arose from one seed of love.

We all start this life as seeds of infinite potential.

If we want our life to be beautiful, we need to cultivate the soil in which we land.

If we want to shape our lives and see our futures we need to look to the seeds we are sowing now, *humility, gratitude, peace.*

If we want to be free, we must compost the most persistent weeds: regret, fear, doubt.

To the Body

❧ *Seed of Potential* ☙

This aptly named pose is a comforting way to start your class. In the embryonic form of the pose, we become seeds of infinite potential. By squeezing our legs into ourselves we soften our external husks.

This practice imitates the shape of a seed with Wind Relief pose variations.

YOUR PERFECTION
Take the pose of a child.

Settle into your mat and wrap your arms around your knees like a swaddled baby.

Rest your head to the floor, lessen the lines of concern between the eyes.

Relax your jaw.

Feel yourself grounding into the earth arms of the Great Mother herself.

Like a rounded seed, in this pose, you carry the potential for all of your life.

You carry all of the elements and sparks of stars.

You carry hope and desire, grace and significance.

In this posture, remember your perfection, beauty, and worthiness.

HALF SEED

1. Lie on your back.
2. Hug your right knee into your chest.
3. Extend your left leg towards the front of your mat.
4. Inhale, hover your left leg off the floor a few centimetres.
5. Exhale, lower your leg.
6. Repeat for five breaths, then switch sides.

SEED BREATHES

1. Lie on your back.
2. Bend your knees towards your chest.
3. Place your hands on your kneecaps.
4. Inhale and lengthen your spine as you move your knees away a little.
5. Exhale, squeeze your knees in.
6. Repeat for four or five rounds.

SEED CIRCLES

1. Lie on your back.
2. Bend your knees in towards your chest.
3. Place your hands on your kneecaps.
4. Make clockwise circles with your knees.

SEED CURLS

1. Lie on your back.
2. Bend your knees towards your chest.
3. Inhale, lengthen your spine along the floor.
4. Exhale, lift your head, neck, and shoulders towards your knees as if you want to kiss them.
5. Repeat steps 3 and 4 five times.

BABY SEED

1. Roll onto your side.
2. Bend your knees and bring them as high up into your chest as possible.

SEATED SEED

1. Come to a seated posture.
2. Bend your knees and place your feet on the floor.
3. Wrap your arms around your shins.
4. Bow your head to your knees.

Seed of Potential

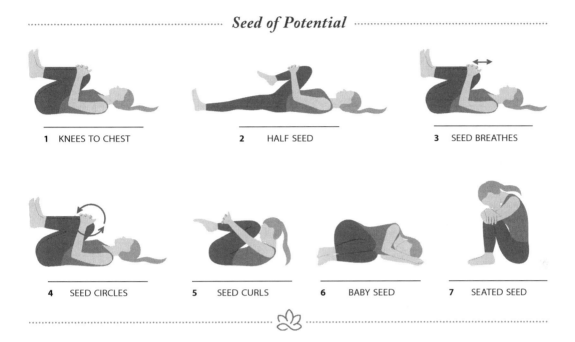

1 KNEES TO CHEST	**2** HALF SEED	**3** SEED BREATHES
4 SEED CIRCLES	**5** SEED CURLS	**6** BABY SEED **7** SEATED SEED

Teaching Notes

Parvana: air or wind

Mukta: freedom, liberate or release

Pawanmuktasana: Wind Relieving pose. In this version of the pose the head is lifted to the knees.

✦ Pawanmuktasana is also a series of small mindful movements to increase circulation and bring mobility to the joints. The set of exercises is recommended for those with impaired mobility, inflammation of the joints, or before practices such as yin yoga. As well as having specific physical benefits, the series is also said to stimulate and move energy throughout the body.

✦ These seed of potential poses are good warm-ups for Child's pose or can be done as alternatives to Child's pose.

✦ Students may enjoy rocking side-to-side or up and down their spine from Wind Relief pose.

CHILD

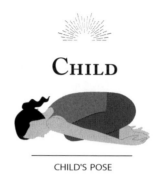

CHILD'S POSE

You are a child of the universe, no less than the trees and the stars;
you have a right to be here.

MAX EHRMANN, 'DESIDERATA'

To the Mind

Bala: child

Balasana: Child's pose

Themes: beginning again, wonder, qualities of a child, finding ease, original goodness

BENEFITS

+ lengthens and stretches the spine and compresses the feet, ankles, and belly

+ pressure on the stomach makes it easier to feel the breath in the back of the body

+ compressing the stomach aids digestion

+ calming, inwards, reflective posture

To the Heart

ORIGINAL GOODNESS

One of the teachings of Buddhism is of Original Goodness. When we look at someone and see behind their eyes, their posture, we look to what is inherently good in that person, what is pure, what is unbroken. When we cast our eyes like this, we can see someone's true spirit or Buddha nature. This childlike approach of seeing everyone and everything for their innate goodness, or more importantly, accepting ourselves as we are rather than our outward appearances, can be remembered in the beautiful pose of a child.

To the Body

❧ *Spark of the Divine* ❧

Below is a series of Child's pose variations to sprinkle throughout your class.

COME AS YOU ARE

Take your posture in the cocoon of Child's pose.

Feel the primary curve of your spine as if it were still in the womb, comfortable, at ease, floating in life.

Drop your weight into the mat, your skin, your bones.

Come as you are.

Drop your worries, your troubles.

At this moment everything is okay.

In this shape, remember your innate goodness.

Your purity.

Your Buddha nature.

CHILD'S POSE

1. Bring your knees together.
2. Sit on your calves and bring your seat to your heels. Use a blanket under your feet or your knees if kneeling is uncomfortable.
3. Wrap your hands down by your sides.

EXTENDED CHILD'S POSE

1. Bring your knees apart and your toes to touch.
2. Lay your body over your knees.
3. Stretch your arms out to the front of the mat.

ANJALI CHILD

1. Come into Child's pose.
2. Bring your elbows to the floor.
3. Bend your elbows; join your palms in Anjali.
4. Fold your palms behind the nape of your neck.

BOUND CHILD

1. Bring your knees together and press your seat to your heels.
2. Bring your hands out in front of you to the floor.
3. Wrap your right hand behind your back, make a fist, and circle your wrist.
4. Swap: bring your left hand behind your back, make wrist circles.
5. Wrap both arms behind your back.
6. Interlace your hands.
7. Press down on your sacrum and spread across your low back.

HUGGING CHILD

1. Come into Child's pose with your knees apart and your toes touching.
2. Thread your arms between your legs and grasp the inner arches of your feet.
3. Turn your face to one side.

CHILD'S TWIST

1. Come into Child's pose with your knees apart and your toes touching.
2. Thread your right arm under your chest and to the left.
3. Turn your head to the left.
4. Repeat on the other side.

LATERAL CHILD

1. Come into Child's pose with your knees apart and your toes touching.

2. Spread your arms out in front.

3. Keep your hips in line and move your upper body to the right.

4. Stretch more through your left arm.

5. Repeat on the other side.

Spark of the Divine

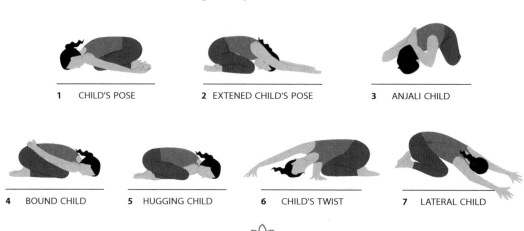

1 CHILD'S POSE   2 EXTENED CHILD'S POSE   3 ANJALI CHILD

4 BOUND CHILD   5 HUGGING CHILD   6 CHILD'S TWIST   7 LATERAL CHILD

Teaching Notes

+ Warm up for Child's pose with Supine Knees to Chest pose either single or double legs.

+ Some people have difficulty with breathing if their belly is compressed. Opening into a wide leg posture can bring more space into the pose.

+ If the head doesn't touch the ground or feels like it is plastered to the ground, a bolster or blanket under the head may alleviate this feeling.

+ The tops of the feet can feel compressed for some students. Offer a blanket to go under the feet.

+ To stretch out feet between Child's pose variations, try Down Dog or Broken Toe pose, where you sit on your flexed toes.

+ For a variety of reasons students may not get their seat to their heels. Offer a rolled blanket for the backs of the knees for comfort or to do Supine Knees to Chest pose.

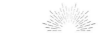

BUDDHA BABY

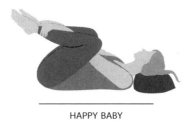

HAPPY BABY

*Happiness is a perfume you cannot pour on others
without getting some on yourself.*

RALPH WALDO EMERSON

To the Mind

Ananda: happy, bliss, blissful, joyous, divine joy, pleasure

Bala: baby

Ananda Balasana: Happy Baby pose

Themes: finding pleasure, sharing success, happiness, mudita

BENEFITS

✦ gently opens inner legs, groins, hamstrings

✦ decompresses the sacrum

✦ massages the back of the body and stimulates the kidneys

✦ allows for compression into the belly and digestive organs

To the Heart

Mudita: unselfish joy, delight in what others have accomplished, being pleased for others' good fortune and success

Mudita is the Buddhist terminology for joy, one of the four *Brahma-vihara* (the abodes of Brahma) along with the virtues of compassion, equanimity, and loving-kindness.

Mudita is to feel unquestionable joy for our life, for what we have, and more importantly, for the success and attainments of others.

One of the obstacles to unselfish joy is comparison. When we look at what others own, how they look, or what they have achieved, it is easy to feel a scarcity that soon dims the light of our internal joy.

But happiness and joy are infinite, and our personal joy holds hands with the collective joy. If we are happy for another, as the Dalai Lama said, there are more chances for happiness than if we are only joyful for ourselves.

To the Body

❧ *Buddha Baby* ☙

Happy Baby and her variations are a comforting way to start or end a class.

Come into Happy Baby, the pose of infinite bliss and the joy of one thousand summers.
Rock side-to-side, tap into the wellspring of happiness that is your birthright.
You were born into this world without deficit and with the capacity for universal happiness.
Know as you rock here that there is no container for this joy unless you give it one.
May you know happiness.
May you feel joy.
May you share this with everyone who walks with you on your path today and all days.

ROCK THE CRADLE

1. Start in Supine Twist with your knees to the right.
2. Open your left leg to the ceiling while keeping your right leg where it is.
3. As you open your left leg, at some point your right leg will start to move up and over to the left.
4. Move slowly, letting your left leg lead.
5. End up in Supine Twist to the left.
6. Move back and forth between sides.

HALF HAPPY BABY

1. Straighten your left leg, and bend your right leg at the knee.
2. Catch hold of your right foot.
3. Pull your right foot with your hand, so your knee moves to your ribs and your foot faces the sky.
4. Repeat on the other side.

HAPPY BABY MODIFICATION

1. Bring the inside edges of your feet together.
2. Catch hold of both your feet between your knees.
3. Pull your feet towards you and widen your knees.

HAPPY BABY

1. Bend your knees towards your outer ribs.
2. Catch hold of your right and left feet with each hand.
3. Point the soles of your feet towards the sky. Relax your knees in the direction of your outer ribs.
4. Lengthen your tailbone forwards.

HAPPY BABY BOLSTER

1. Lay a bolster on your belly.
2. Hook your feet on top of one another around the bolster.
3. Cross one ankle over the other.
4. Hug the bolster with your arms.

YIN BABY

1. Move to a wall.
2. Lie on your back.
3. Separate your legs.
4. Bend your knees and place the soles of your feet on the wall.

Buddha Baby

1   ROCK THE CRADLE

2   HALF HAPPY BABY

3   HAPPY BABY MODIFICATION

4   HAPPY BABY

5   HAPPY BABY BOLSTER

6   YIN BABY

Teaching Notes

+ Have a strap for students for Half Happy Baby. Place the strap around the sole of the foot and hold the strap in the same side hand.

+ The feet, ankles, or backs of the knees can be held. Some students prefer to hold their toes or the inside of their feet.

+ The knees can come to the outside of the ribs or sit inside the rib line.

+ A block or blanket under the head may be supportive for those students whose chins jut upwards.

+ A blanket under the low back will support and encourage students to let their sacrum be heavy towards the ground.

+ Rocking in poses has a calming, soothing effect on the nervous system.

CROCODILE

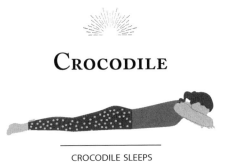

CROCODILE SLEEPS

May I live like the lotus, at home in the muddy water.

ANONYMOUS

To the Mind

Makra: crocodile

Makrasana: Crocodile pose

Themes: breathing, stress relief, letting go, overcoming fear, second chakra

BENEFITS

+ great starting pose for teaching diaphragmatic breathing

+ relaxes the nervous system, relieves stress and tension

+ brings a gentle compression into the low back, which makes it an excellent alternative to Cobra

+ with the knee up, it releases one side of the sacrum

To the Heart

THE CROCODILE LIVES IN THE MURKY WATERS

In Hindu mythology, the crocodile is the mount for the goddess Ganga who is the guardian of the sacred waters of the Ganges. The Ganges are revered for their ability to heal and release people from the cycle of birth and death. Aspirants enter the water for purification and healing. The water is murky, which symbolises what we can't see in the depths.

As a primitive symbol of fear, Ganga rides the back of the crocodile as if to say *I feel what is difficult and what frightens me, but to grow I need to move through this to overcome my demons.*

We all have our inner battles that lie at the depths of our beings. It seems more comfortable to let things lie, to look away or to keep things hidden, but eventually, what is hidden will want to ascend.

To the Body

◇ *At Home in the Murky Waters* ◆

BREATHE WITH THE CROCODILE

Crocodile posture is perfect for practising diaphragmatic breathing. In our day-to-day life, we tend to breathe unconsciously, without thought. When we bring attention to our breath, we bring awareness to what lies in the unconscious mind. Like a dormant crocodile lying in murky water, we then start to bring up other thoughts and emotions that lie beneath the surface.

Lie down, relax. Feel your belly spread and soften like silk on the floor.

Start to take some long slow breaths into your centre as if you were trying to light up your personal solar system.

Without force, feel the steady build of pressure as the diaphragm moves down on the inhale, and the release and rise on the exhale.

Become more sensitive to where the breath is going into your body.

Feel yourself fill up three-dimensionally—back, sides, and front—as if you were breathing into a balloon.

Keep breathing like this; in, out.

Sense your diaphragm move in unison with your breath. Up and down like the giant sweep of a manta ray's wings, without disturbing the water.

Take in what you need.

What does it feel like to be so sensitive towards yourself?

Keep pouring your awareness into the next few breaths.

DIAPHRAGMATIC BREATHING

1. Lie in one of the versions of Crocodile. Lying on the belly to breathe helps bring the feeling of the breath into the back and sides of your body.

2. Feel your chest and upper body weighted to the floor.

3. Bring your attention to your mid-low back to where the diaphragm straddles your body.

4. Take a long slow breath in and feel your belly swell and press into the earth. Exhale slowly. Take five long, slow breaths here, sensing the compression and release with each breath in and out.

5. Let the breath spread to the back of your body for five slow breaths.

6. Take your breath to the sides of your body at the mid-low back. Feel as if your breath is spreading your ribs and opening your sides.

CROCODILE SLEEPS

1. Lie on your belly.

2. Fold your arms.

3. Rest your forehead on your arms.

4. Let your legs relax.

5. Make gentle side-to-side movements with your pelvis.

BROKEN WINGS

1. Lie on your belly.

2. Cross your right arm under your chest to the left.

3. Lay your left arm at a right angle under your forehead.

4. Rest your forehead on your left arm.

5. Let the weight of your body fall onto your right arm.

6. Repeat on the other side.

CROCODILE YAWNS

1. Lie on your belly.

2. Bring your arms by your sides, palms up or down.

3. Turn your face to one side.

CROCODILE BRIDGE

1. Place a bolster lengthways on your mat.

2. Lay your torso, from your pubic bone to your breastbone, on the bolster.

3. Place your head and shoulders on the floor off the bolster.

CROCODILE ARCH

1. Lie on your belly.

2. Rest your forehead on your arms.

3. Hook your right knee up to 90 degrees.

4. Crab walk your body to the right, so there is an arch on the left side of your body.

At home in the Murky Waters

1 CROCODILE SLEEPS

2 BROKEN WINGS

3 CROCODILE YAWNS

4 CROCODILE BRIDGE

5 CROCODILE ARCH

Teaching Notes

✦ Crocodile gently stimulates the second chakra region. Svadhisthana is home to our powerful urges, our creativity, our deeply held emotions, our habits and fears. Kundalini shakti lies here.

✦ Resting the third eye centre on your arms also stimulates ajna, or the third eye chakra.

✦ Crocodile pose puts gentle pressure on the belly, which stimulates digestion. From here you can lead into more belly compression with blankets or compression in Child's pose or Knees to Chest pose.

✦ The home of the crocodile is the water, so this pose naturally fits in with the water theme.

✦ The crocodile lives happily on the land or in the water, representing both steadiness and flow, first and second chakra.

✦ The lotus is a flower that is at home in the mud. Consider using this analogy with Padma (lotus) mudra.

FULL PROSTRATION

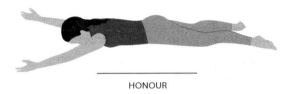

HONOUR

As you rise with the morning sun think to yourself
what a privilege it is to be alive, to breathe, to think, to enjoy, to love.
MARCUS AURELIUS

To the Mind

Nam: bow

Prana: life force

Pranam: respecting, honouring, surrendering, paying homage to life

Themes: offering, respect, paying tribute, counting your blessings, honouring your past, ishvara pranidhana (alignment with a higher power)

BENEFITS:

+ connects us fully to the earth and has a grounding effect

+ helps us lay down our burdens or worries

+ relaxes and de-stresses

To the Heart

When we perform prostrations of any kind, we observe the five-thousand-year-old tradition known as yoga. Originally, laying the belly flat on the floor and stretching the arms forwards came after the more modern Chaturanga or Four-Limbed Staff pose, which is most frequently performed in Sun Salutation.

In Tibetan, the word prostration is translated as 'to sweep away' (anything that stands in our path), so that we may receive blessings. When we lay the points of our body down—feet, hands, belly, head—in this primal ritual, we honour the tradition and appreciate its value. This embodied practice of respect and worship for our life and all life can be felt most intimately in full Pranam.

To the Body

⤙ *Honour* ⤚

Honour your life.
The comings and goings.
The falling apart and coming together.

Honour your lineage.
What was handed to you and what you will pass to others is your gift to the world.

Honour who you are.
What you know and don't know.
Your strengths and vulnerabilities.
All of these make you beautiful in some way.
Honour your feelings.
The sadness, the bites of anger.
The knife tips of fear.
The joy!

Honour the beauty and symbiosis of your relationships.
Some of them will help you thrive.
Some will dismantle you into jigsaw pieces.
All of them will teach you.

Whatever you came into this world with, it is yours.
It is loyal.
It loves you.
And it is waiting for you to
honour it.

PRANAM

1. Lie down on your mat.

2. Feel your belly spread onto the belly of the earth.

3. Rest your forehead down. Let it be heavy.

4. Stretch your arms out as a symbolic gesture of appreciation and gratitude for this life.

5. Honour yourself.

Honour

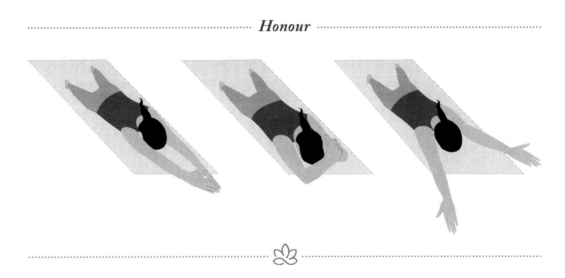

Teaching Notes

+ Pranam can be performed with the arms outstretched and palms joined together, with the elbows bent and hands joined in Anjali mudra, with the hands stretched out and the arms shoulder distance apart, or fold the arms and rest the forehead on your arms.

+ Stay a few breaths in each Pranam to experience the connection to the earth and to embody the practice as an offering or to lay down your troubles into the great Mother Earth.

+ See also ishvara pranidhana for more ideas on the theme of devotion.

CONSTRUCTIVE REST

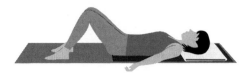

To the mind that is still the whole universe surrenders.

BUDDHA

To the Mind

Shava: corpse

Mrtasana: death

Constructive Rest: is an alternative to Savasana

Themes: letting go, core values, rest, Savasana or the Rebound in yin yoga practices

BENEFITS:

+ Calming for the nervous system
+ Helps reset the posture
+ Relaxes tension in the spine
+ Helps calm breathing
+ Soothes the psoas muscle

To the Heart

The sacrum is a wide bone at the base of the spine. It comes from the Latin word *sacred*. No one is sure why this bone is sacred. Maybe it is because it is a protector of the organs that produce life. Maybe because it is the foundation for the elegant spine, or that in its power it is the last bone to decay after death.

Things that are sacred are those that are worthy of attention, lie close to our bones, and those that need protecting or preserving. They give us strength and are our core values—the values that will drive our life.

If you have never taken the time to think about your core values or what is true for you, the non-negotiables, the things you will stand up for, now is the time.

To the Body

☙ *Learning to Let Go* ❧

Come into Constructive Rest.

Spread your back body on the floor, take up as much space as you need.

Anchor your sacrum to the earth.

Imagine it opening and spreading like a Japanese fan.

Close your eyes.

Be here.

Trust.

Take a moment, get still.

Place one hand on your heart; this is the sacred abode of all you hold true.

What do you place on the altar of your heart?

What do you want to preserve and protect and hold close?

Envision it, stow it there, make it sacred.

This love letter to yourself can never be taken away.

CONSTRUCTIVE REST POSE

1. Lie on your mat; you may like to place a blanket down for extra comfort.

2. Bend your knees and place your feet on the floor hip-distance apart.

3. If you have lower back issues you can let your knees fall inwards to touch.

4. Turn your palms up.

5. Rest your arms on the floor. If your shoulders are tight, place a folded blanket under each arm.

BOUND CONSTRUCTIVE REST

1. Fold a blanket into a square and place it at the base of your mat.

2. Make a loop with a strap big enough to wrap around your thighs. Slide this up your thighs and lie down.

3. Bend your knees and place your feet on the blanket.

4. Adjust the strap so your legs are resting in the loop.

5. Place an eye pillow over your eyes.

6. Fold your arms over your chest.

SUPPORTED CONSTRUCTIVE REST

1. Fold a blanket several times to form a pillow big enough for your hips and sacrum to rest on.
2. Lie down.
3. Bend your knees and lift up your hips.
4. Slide the blanket or support under your hips.

RESTORATIVE CONSTRUCTIVE REST

1. Place a chair on your mat.
2. Place a blanket over the chair seat if you prefer.
3. Lie down and swing your legs up onto the chair so the crooks of your knees are lined up with the front of the seat.
4. Rest your head on a folded blanket.
5. Spread your arms wide.

Learning to Let Go

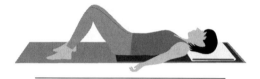

1   CONSTRUCTIVE REST

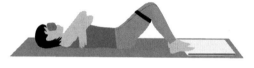

2   BOUND CONSTRUCTIVE REST

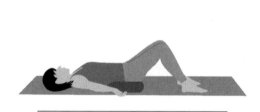

3   SUPPORTED CONSTRUCTIVE REST

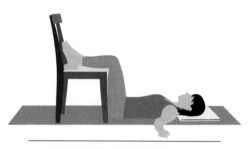

4   RESTORATIVE CONSTRUCTIVE REST

Teaching Notes

✦ Contructive Rest can be done at the beginning or end of a class or as a transition pose.

✦ It is deeply relaxing as the spine is supported and it allows the psoas muscles to drop and release.

✦ It can be used as an alternative to Savasana or may suit those who find lying with their legs straight uncomfortable.

✦ This pose can accompany yoga nidra practices.

SUPPORTED FISH

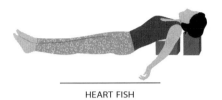

HEART FISH

Man sees in the world what he carries in his heart.
GOETHE

To the Mind

Matsya: fish

Matsyasana: Fish pose—backbend

Themes: fifth chakra, speaking your truth, loving all parts of yourself, finding your strengths, fourth chakra or heart opening

BENEFITS

+ stretches the front line of the body, including the muscles between the ribs, the belly, and the hip flexors.

+ relaxes the shoulder heads and lifts the back of the body into the front of the body.

+ expands and opens the lungs, which assists in breathing.

+ opens the throat.

+ is a mild inversion.

+ often used as a counterpose for Shoulder Stand.

+ Supported Fish or Heart Bridge in yin yoga is an opening posture that negates a day of hunching forwards.

+ opens the front of the throat, letting out the unsaid.

To the Heart

THE EVOLUTION OF THE FISH

Long before you came into this world, your heart had its vinyasa. From a single chamber to two chambers to three, it evolved—fish to frog to snake—before finally settling into the human four-chambered form. The heart's four faces are compassion, empathy, joy, and equanimity.

One hundred thousand beats a day tap a rhythm responding to your movement and your emotions.

This life pulses through you, animating your practice; without this drumbeat, there would be no life. Each beat is a note, and you are the note-taker in your most extraordinary composition.

To the Body

To Love All Parts

A tender way to start any class, this posture brings focus to the heart, the fist-sized organ that lies slightly to the left and behind the breastbone.

You can combine any of the versions of Supported Fish Pose with Heart Tapping.

Your heart
has the capacity to hold the smallest of things or the uncountable.
This container of love beats for you, a steady sentinel, without asking for a thing.
It firstly beats for itself, feeding itself with blood and then feeding the other organs.
This act of self-kindness, self-compassion, animates our life
and is a gentle reminder
to act from the heart.

HEART TAPPING

Heart Tapping brings awareness to the heart space but also is said to affect the thymus gland, which lies in this region. Palpating this area may help boost immunity.

1. Choose one of the postures below.

2. Bring your fingertips and thumb together (also known as Mukula mudra) and tap on your breastbone gently around your sternum.

3. Choose your rhythm and intensity as you move up and down the bony plate of your chest.

FLOATING FISH

1. Fold two blankets, one for under your head and one for under your mid-to-low back. Make about three half folds. You may need to adjust the head blanket and make it a little higher by folding it one more time lengthways.

2. Place the blankets on your mat with a gap of about fifteen to twenty centimetres, enough room for your shoulders and arms.

3. Lie down and place one blanket under your head and one under your back.

4. Open your arms out to right angles.

HEART FISH

1. Place one block on the mat on the mid to high setting and another block lengthways on the mat mid to low setting. This bottom block should be under your mid-back, not your low back.

2. Lie down on the mat. Place the weight of your head on the high block and your mid-back on the low block.

3. Open your arms up.

4. Choose your leg variations: bent legs, straight legs, diamond-shape legs.

FISH IN A BROOK

1. Fold a blanket to support your upper back and head, about two to three folds.

2. Fold another blanket into a smaller cylinder shape, which will go under your knees. You can also use a bolster.

3. Lie down with your head and shoulders on the blanket and your knees draping over the support.

FISH OUT OF WATER

1. Take a bolster and turn it lengthways on your mat.

2. Sit down on your mat with the bolster in the small of your back.

3. Lay your torso and head on the bolster, so they are supported.

To Love All Parts

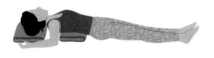

1   FLOATING FISH

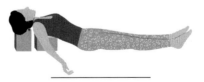

2   HEART FISH

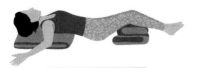

3   FISH IN A BROOK

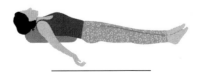

4 FISH OUT OF WATER

Teaching Notes

+ Fish pose is often used as a counterpose for Shoulder Stand.

+ Some students report feeling nauseous with their head below their neck in Fish. Prop up students' heads higher than their hearts to alleviate any discomfort.

+ If you chose to work with Fish pose or water as a theme you may like to add in the pose Matsyendrasana or Half Lord of the Fishes pose. This pose is a twist and has several variations. Matsyendra is often attributed as one of the founders of hatha yoga.

THE STORY OF MATSYENDRA

Matsyendra was born under an inauspicious star, so his parents cast him into the water where a fish swallowed him.

One day as this fish was bathing in the shallows of the river, he heard the teachings of Shiva, who was imparting his knowledge of yoga to Parvati, his wife. The fish absorbed the teachings of yoga and left the river to spread this knowledge.

Matsyendra transformed himself from an unwanted baby to the 'father of yoga.'

This allegory is a reminder that by casting out the parts of us that are unwanted, we also submerge our potential.

We can shift our weaknesses into something powerful.
Our darkness is also our light.
Our shortcomings can bear gifts.
Our blind sides are an opportunity to learn.

Thunderbolt

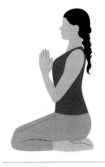

VAJRASANA

I saw the angel in the marble and carved until I set him free.
Michelangelo

To the Mind

Vajra: thunderbolt, diamond, an instrument of battle

Vajrasana: Thunderbolt pose or Seiza. In Japanese culture, sitting in Seiza is seen as a sign of courtesy while attending tea ceremonies or cultural events. When you bow forwards with your hands outstretched it is physical embodiment of apology. Seiza is also used for meditation.

Themes: strengths, adversity, trust, belief in yourself, fearlessness

BENEFITS

✦ compression of the legs increases blood flow to the digestive organs.

✦ sitting upright strengthens the spine and restores its natural postural curves

✦ encourages stability in the body, which in turn can have a calming effect on the mind

To the Heart

The diamond is formed in the earth under pressure and then shaped into something of beauty and value.

It is rubbed raw to conquer itself, to break through the pressure of life so it can be brought into the light.

We practice to bring ourselves up from the ground into the diamond light. And it is in this light that our troubles, our fears, our inner critics will be quelled.

To the Body

❧ *Diamond in the Rough* ☙

VAJRA

1. Sit back onto your calves or a block.
2. Take a moment to find balance left-to-right, front-to-back. This posture is called Vajra.

DIAMOND CAT-COW

1. Sit on the block or your calves.
2. Place your hands on your knees and begin to arch and flex your spine.
3. Make these gentle Cat-Cow movements and feel the ripple of energy move through your torso.

DIAMOND BIND

1. Sit on a block or your shins.
2. Interlace your fingers and reach up for the sky.

DIAMOND TWIST

1. Sit on a block or your shins and turn your torso to the left.
2. Bring your right hand over your left knee and place your left hand on the floor or a block behind you.
3. Repeat this twist to the right side.

DIAMOND COW FACE

1. Sit on a block or your shins.
2. Bring your right arm above your head, and bend your elbow to place your right hand at the back of your neck.
3. Take your left arm out to the side in line with your shoulder.
4. Turn your palm back, so your thumb faces the ground.
5. Wrap your left arm behind your back.
6. Bind your left hand to your right with a strap or your hands.
7. Repeat on the other side.

VAJRA PADMA MUDRA:
UNSHAKEABLE TRUST

This mudra builds an unshakable belief, confidence, and courage in yourself.

The diamond is hard and unbreakable, the thunderbolt unstoppable and fearless. When you have unshakable trust in who you are, you take on these qualities and become a force that can overcome obstacles with ease.

The hands form a web to symbolise interconnectedness.

The mudra is a show of your power, that even in life's most difficult situations, there is a part of you that is whole and ready to rise to the challenge.

To perform Vajra Padma mudra, interlace your fingers to the webbing; leave your thumbs free. Place the mudra on your heart.

Diamond in the Rough

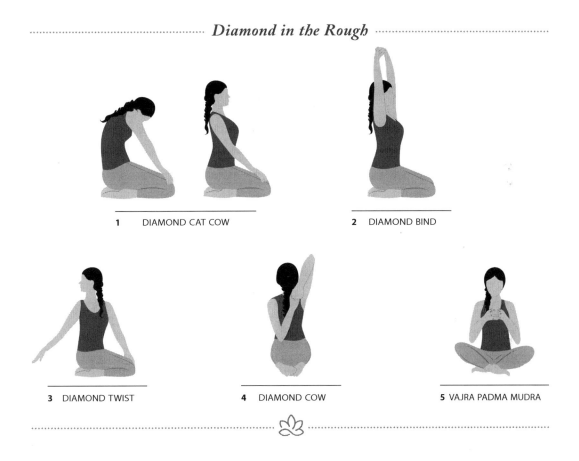

1   DIAMOND CAT COW

2   DIAMOND BIND

3   DIAMOND TWIST

4   DIAMOND COW

5 VAJRA PADMA MUDRA

Teaching Notes

+ Vajrasana is the cousin of Virasana. Vira means hero. In Vajrasana you sit on your calves whereas in Virasana you sit between your legs.

+ Child's pose is sometimes called Adho Mukha Virasana, or Downward Facing Hero.

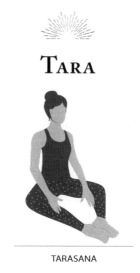

TARA

TARASANA

If you want others to be happy, practice compassion.
If you want to be happy, practice compassion.

DALAI LAMA

To the Mind

Tara: star, the deity of compassion and support, saviour

Tarasana: Star pose

Themes: compassion, suffering or loss, grieving, love and care, being guided or supported

BENEFITS

+ seated Forward Fold variation opens the backline of the body
+ lengthens the groin and inner thighs
+ nourishes and stimulates the internal organs, increasing blood flow
+ opens the root chakra and sacral chakra

To the Heart

In Buddhism, the goddess Tara has twenty-one colours, but it is mainly her white and green hues that form the basis of meditations that invoke her energy. She is also known as the female Buddha.

TARA THE PROTECTOR

Green Tara is the protector who watches over us on our physical and spiritual journey through this life. This saviour will usher us from danger and encourage us on our paths, helping us overcome the most difficult of situations. She acts quickly to be by our sides. Her seven eyes—on her hands, feet, face, and third eye—represent her watchful nature over all of life. Her eyes shine out like a lighthouse so she can see more clearly and so that others who need guidance can see in the dark. Like a captain of a pilot boat, she guides you through unchartered territory, carrying you to shore.

If we look with bright eyes, we will see the signposts. A bird fluttering around our shoulder, a reoccurring dream, synchronicity, or ideas that keep tapping on our shoulder—Tara is guiding us.

TARA AND COMPASSION

The white and pure radiance of Tara symbolises compassion and peace. It is said her heart for all sentient beings is more potent than a mother's love for their children. People pray to her for life-long healing and to help those wounded in the body or mind.

Compassion comes from the word 'compi' meaning to suffer with or to hold another's suffering. This basic human instinct to care for others is deeply rooted and can be quickly mobilised should we hear someone's cries for help.

Self-compassion is to hold your suffering with tenderness, as you would cradle a friend's pain. It can be a little more difficult to access when we are at the centre of our sadness. Learning how to sit with others' heartbreaks or despair trains us to be able to practice compassion for ourselves.

When we wake up and learn to see that we are all in this together, that we all suffer in the same way, that we are part of humanity and its suffering, then we can open our hearts to tending the wounds of ourselves and others.

The Buddhist tradition teaches *tonglen*, a tool for relieving the suffering of others. In today's world, it is easy to get immobilised by devastating events. This practice reminds us not to turn away from the pain of others or of ourselves but to breathe in the hurt and breathe out something more expansive and healing. It is through this practice that we collectively share the individual burden. Through this sharing of empathy and compassion comes healing.

THE TALE OF THE MUSTARD SEEDS

Kisa Gotami was born poor but married into a wealthy family. She gave birth to a son who lost his life as a toddler. The distraught mother was sent to Buddha to ask him to bring her son back to life.

Buddha agreed to help her. He told her that she must go door to door in the village to get some mustard seeds. There was one proviso, and that was the seeds must come from a house that had never known death.

Kisa went door to door but couldn't find any villagers who had not felt her pain through loss of a loved one. She slowly began to realise that she was not alone in her suffering, and death is a natural part of life. She began to see that she hadn't been singled out to receive hurt. This realisation helped her befriend her situation, so she was able to let her son go.

Although the pain of losing a loved one, especially a young life, is never easy, this story reminds us of the impermanence of life. As the unripe fruit falls from the tree and the ripe ones get eaten, nature understands this process. When Kisa connected with others' pain and heartbreak, she began to understand the universality of life and was able to find a way through her grief.

When we step out of our pain even for a brief minute, we too can remember that we are not alone in our losses.

To the Body

❧ Tara's Dance ☙

HAPPY BABY VARIATION

1. Lie on your back for this Happy Baby variation.
2. Hug your knees into your chest.
3. Grasp your feet in your right and left hands.
4. Pull your feet to your belly.
5. Let your knees fall out to the side to make a diamond shape.

OUTSTRETCHED STAR

1. Lie on your back.
2. Join the soles of your feet together and let your knees fall out wide to make a diamond shape.
3. Reach your arms overhead and stretch them away from your pelvis.

BUTTERFLY FLAPS ITS WINGS

1. Come to a seated position.
2. Join the soles of your feet together and let your knees fall out wide.
3. Hold your feet together in your hands.
4. Move your knees up and down, slowly then more quickly, flapping them like wings.

TARA TWIST

1. Come to a seated position.
2. Join the soles of your feet together and let your knees fall out wide.
3. Twist to your left.
4. Place your right hand over your left knee and your left hand behind you on the floor.
5. Repeat on the other side.

TARA SIDE BEND

1. Come to a seated position.
2. Join the soles of your feet together and let your knees fall out wide.
3. Twist to your left.
4. Place your right hand on your outer left knee.
5. Lean your body to the right.
6. Reach your left hand to the sky.
7. Repeat on the other side.

TARA FOLD

1. Come to a seat.
2. Join the soles of your feet together and let your knees fall out wide.
3. Fold forwards over your legs.

Tara's Dance

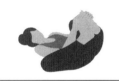

1 HAPPY BABY VARIATION

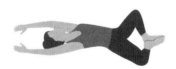

2 OUTSTRETCHED STAR

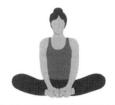

3 BUTTERFLY FLAPS ITS WINGS

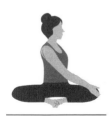

4 TARA TWIST

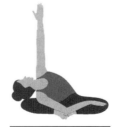

5 TARA SIDE BEND

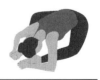

6 TARA FOLD

Teaching Notes

+ Tara pose is a gentle, receptive posture to begin any practice.

+ The pose can be done seated or lying down.

+ In yin yoga practices, it is named Butterfly.

+ Tarasana differs from Bound Angle pose. In Tarasana the knees are bent at 90 degrees, so the shape of the legs forms a diamond. In Bound Angle the heels are pulled closer to the groins and the soles of the feet are turned more upwards.

SUPINE BOUND ANGLE

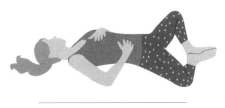

SUPINE BOUND ANGLE

You can search throughout the entire universe for someone who is more deserving of your love and affection than you are yourself, and that person is not to be found anywhere. You yourself, as much as anybody in the entire universe, deserve your love and affection.

BUDDHA

To the Mind

Baddha: bound

Kona: angle

Baddha Konasana: Bound Angle pose

Supta: reclined or supine

Supta Baddha Konasana: supine Bound Angle pose
Bound Angle, a cousin of Tarasana, is also called Cobbler's pose. In India, cobblers would place the shoe they were working on between their feet to hold it in place. It differs from Tarasana in that the feet are drawn closer to the groins and ideally the soles of the feet turn upwards.
Supine Bound Angle is a beautiful pose to start dropping into your body, connecting to your breath and being reminded of the practice of self-love.

Themes: your perfection, being content with who you are, exploring the meaning of self-improvement, internal goodness

BENEFITS

+ stretches through the inner leg line into the groin

+ brings focus to the digestive and reproductive systems

+ supine version is an excellent posture to acclimatise to belly breathing

+ opens the front line of the body and stimulates lung and heart qi

+ with one hand on your heart, it brings attention to the physical heart and its qualities of love, and self-love

To the Heart

Sometimes we are so intent on improving ourselves that we forget to take time out to be okay with who and where we are in life. If we continually strive to push forwards, we may become depleted in the impossible search to be good enough.

When we are too busy trying to alter our external landscapes, we can easily forget that yoga is the process of uncovering our internal goodness, that it is a journey towards wholeness. It is about loving all parts of ourselves.

If we push away or try to reject the parts of us that feel like dislike, shame, or failure, we separate from this wholeness.

The first place to start with self-love is to remember your worthiness.

To the Body

ꙷ Supine Bound Angle ꙷ

Lie down.

Settle here.

Kiss the soles of your feet together and let your knees turn out left and right to form a diamond shape.

Place one hand on your all-loving, forgiving heart, and one on your belly brain, the well of knowing and sensing.

Start to breathe into your hands.

Let your breath and touch be a conduit to a greater awareness within.

Now dive deeper under the skin and feel inside.
Under your hands is the pulse of life, a place that is untouched and perfect, your north star.

Your heart, your bright leading light, is the part that signed up for this journey.

Your worth is not dependent on how you look or what you do or how much you earn. Your worth is sealed in the vault of your heart. Take heart in knowing your uniqueness and the gifts you bring to this world are of utmost value.

Today, as you move through this practice, may you find appreciation and may you remember your worthiness.

SUPINE BOUND ANGLE

1. Lie on your back.
2. Bring the soles of your feet together to form a diamond shape with your legs. Place a support under your knees if needed.
3. Place one hand on your heart and one hand on your belly.
4. Breathe into your hands.

SUPPORTED BOUND ANGLE

1. Make a large loop in a strap and place it around your low back with the buckle near your lower leg.
2. Place the soles of your feet together.
3. Place a bolster vertical to the small of your back.
4. Loop the strap around your back, over the inside of your knees and around the small toe side of your closed feet.
5. Lay your spine over the bolster.
6. Adjust the strap by pulling on the loose end until the pose feels supported.

Bound Angle

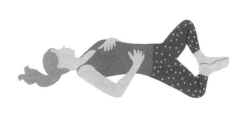

1   SUPINE BOUND ANGLE

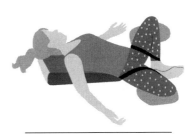

2   SUPPORTED BOUND ANGLE

Teaching Notes

+ Salamba: supported

+ Supine Bound Angle and Supported Bound Angle are also good postures to end a class prior to Savasana.

+ With one hand on the heart and one on the belly, Supine Bound Angle is a sensitive way to practice belly breathing, (the swell of the belly on the inhale).

+ Seated Bound Angle is a gentle way to start a class as it releases the hamstrings which allows the students to bow more readily.

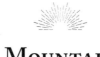

MOUNTAIN

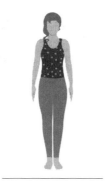

MOUNTAIN POSE

You are not in the mountains. The mountains are in you.

JOHN MUIR

To the Mind

Tada: mountain

Tadasana: Mountain pose

Themes: rising above small grievances, standing tall, Mountain pose as the basis for all postures, confidence, balance, stability

BENEFITS

+ helps postural alignment
+ good spinal alignment allows a freer flow of energy through the body
+ strengthens and tones the lower body
+ helps us tune in to our core stabilisers to balance

To the Heart

Mountain pose, or *Tadasana*, is the blueprint for most yoga poses. When we learn the principles of standing on our own two feet with confidence, this naturally transfers into all the postures of our life or practice.

Mountain pose is a confident way to stand in good alignment. The spine has form and shape and bends like a river, so to stand in Mountain is to stand between bracing and collapse, or equal standing (Samasthiti). When we stand with effort and ease, in balance and stillness, this information highway can sing to all the tributaries that feed off it.

Physically, energetically and spiritually, Mountain pose is the guardian for all our postures both on and off the mat.

To the Body

☽ *Move Like a Mountain* ☾

Mountain pose is a noble way to start a class. The movements below will free up the spine and shift stagnant energy.

> *The birds have vanished into the sky,*
> *And now the last cloud drains away.*
> *We sit together, the mountain and me,*
> *Until only the mountain remains.*
>
> LI PO

STAND TALL
Feel lines of energy run from the navel to the toes and from the navel to the crown.
Press your feet into the riverbed and feel a buoyancy in your chest.
Feel your body as if it is suspended in space and your head almost floating off your shoulders.
Your feet in the earth, your head in the clouds, grounding meets clarity.
You are a mountain, barely marked by wind or rain.

BE YOUR OWN SHERPA
Stand in Mountain pose; make small movements to balance your body evenly.
Front to back.
Top to bottom.
Movement to stillness to peace.
Strength and grace.
When you stand this way, you return home to your energetic blueprint, the conduit between heaven and earth.
In Tadasana can you embody the strength and grace of the mountain within you?

Like climbing the sacred Mount Kailash, when you stand here, you stand on the edge of your spiritual journey.

When you make any pilgrimage, there is so much to learn, and your journey will take many forms.

When the bad weather comes, you will be your own sherpa, guiding your way with conviction.

And when the sun shines, it will light your steady way.

RISE ABOVE

Stand tall in your posture.

Embody the stability and stature of your favourite mountain.

Don't settle for mediocrity.

The way we stand affects the way we feel. When we stand tall, we can rise above ourselves.

So what do you want to rise above today?

Rise above the stories in your head; you are more significant than any narrative.

Rise above the history and the battle wounds. You have already come so far.

Rise above the day-to-day struggles you have with yourself. People are looking to you for how to act.

Hold your face to the sun and let each Ujjayi breath remind you to stand tall and triumphant,

as the mighty Kauri guardians stand, the cornerstones of the forest.

MOUNTAIN POSE TWISTS

1. Stand in Mountain pose.
2. Bring your hands to your heart.
3. Turn your upper body to the right and spread your arms wide at shoulder height.
4. Bring your hands to your heart in Anjali mudra.
5. Turn your body to the left and open your arms.
6. Bring your hands back to your heart.

EMBRACE THE MOUNTAIN

1. Stand in Mountain pose.
2. Inhale, open your arms wide to shoulder height, lift your sternum and arch backwards.
3. Exhale, flex your upper back, and curl your arms inwards as if you were holding a giant beach ball.
4. Inhale, open your arms wide, and extend your upper back into a small backbend.
5. Continue opening and closing your upper spine for five rounds.

SPINAL ROLLS

1. Start in Mountain pose with your arms by your sides.
2. Tuck your chin in towards your chest and roll down one vertebra at a time; your back will be rounded.
3. Imagine your spine is like a stack of beads, and you are peeling them away from each other one at a time.

4. Roll back to standing, one vertebra at a time.

5. Turn your chest to the right and roll down the right leg slowly.

6. Return to Mountain.

7. Turn your chest to the left and roll down your left leg.

8. Unwind slowly back up to Mountain.

9. Roll back down to the floor and stay dangling or move into your vinyasa flow.

AROUND THE MOUNTAIN

1. Stand in Mountain pose and place your right hand over your chest and onto your left shoulder.

2. Cross your left hand onto your right shoulder.

3. Make small circles with your upper back, chest, and head.

4. Try to isolate the upper back in the movement.

Move Like a Mountain

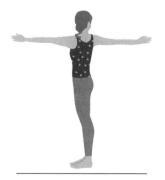

1 MOUNTAIN POSE TWISTS

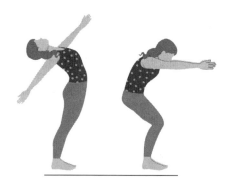

2 EMBRACE THE MOUNTAIN

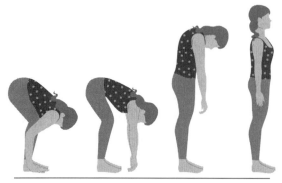

3 SPINAL ROLLS

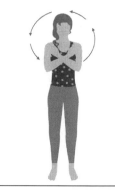

4 AROUND THE MOUNTAIN

Teaching Notes

Urdhva: upwards or lifted

Urdhva Hastasana: Upward Salute pose, usually with the arms and feet apart.

Urdhva Namaskarasana: Upward Prayer pose, the palms of the hands join together above the head with straight arms and the feet are usually together.

+ In the Sun Salutation sequences Mountain pose is often followed with Upward Salute pose or Upward Prayer pose.

+ Balance or equal standing should be found between the left and right sides of the body, the front and back, the crown and feet. When embodying Mountain pose in any pose, can you find equal standing in the organ body? Sense between the two sides of the brain, the ears, the lungs, the kidneys, and the sacrum.

SUPINE TREE

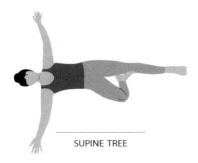

SUPINE TREE

In a forest of a hundred thousand trees, no two leaves are alike.
And no two journeys along the same path are alike.

PAULO COELHO

To the Mind

Vrksa: tree

Vrksasana: Tree pose

Supta: reclined or supine

Supta Vrksasana: reclined Tree pose

Themes: balance, connection, roots to our ancestry and past, support, effort and ease

BENEFITS

+ stretches inner thighs and groins

+ standing versions increase balance and coordination while strengthening the legs

+ relaxes the nervous system

+ calms the mind

To the Heart

The patient, steady tree lives in rhythm with the cycle of life. Many cultures have looked to trees for healing, not only by using parts of the tree for medicine but by bathing in their energy in a practice known in Japan as *shinrin-yoku*, or forest bathing. This practice has been studied for its benefits to our psyche and our soma (physical self), including lowering blood pressure, improving mood, lowering cholesterol, fighting inflammation, and improving mental well-being.[5]

When we walk in the protective canopy and use our senses to engage in the forest, when we engage in conscious connection to the power of the trees, we are practising preventative medicine.

Metaphorically, the standing leg in Tree weights into the earth. This single root connects us to ancestral roots—our lineage, and all those who have walked the path before us.

Just as the roots of live trees spread unseen words of warnings to protect and support the others, when we take the shape of the tree, we can remember the support, protection, and guidance of our community. As we physically tap into the symbiotic energy of the planet with our feet, we become one with a higher source of power that emanates from the foundations of the soil.

To the Body

✷ *Forest Bathing* ✷

This practice uses the wall as support. When we are given a grounded lifeline, we can explore the pose while remaining stable and connected.

SUPINE TREE

Lie down on your back. Draw your left knee out to the side and make the shape of Tree.

As you lie here, feel each bone of your spine press into the clay earth, as if you want to put roots down into the soft land beneath you.

Feel your right leg heavy, like the stump of a fallen tree.

Tap into that place within that is solid, stable, and supportive, like the mighty Tāne Mahuta[6]; make this your anchor.

As you breathe life into your tree, feel the lungs of this land breathe into you.

Remember, you are not alone—you are held here by all the other trees and protected by the shade of the canopy.

---

[5] Qing Li, *Forest Bathing: How Trees Can Help You Find Health and Happiness.* Viking, 2018.

[6] Tāne Mahuta is a giant kauri tree in the Waipoua Forest of Northland Region, New Zealand. Tāne is the God of the forest and birds. One of the oldest trees in the world, it is estimated to be between 1,250 and 2,500 years. It is the largest kauri known to stand today, at 51 metres high and with a circumference of 13.8 metres.

FLOWING TREE

1. Lie with the soles of your feet against the wall.

2. Press your feet evenly into the wall as if you were standing on the ground.

3. As you inhale, draw your right leg up and your hands overhead as if you were doing Tree pose on your back.

4. Exhale, place your right foot back to the wall and your arms by your sides.

5. Repeat several times before changing to the left side.

WILLOW SUPINE

1. Place your right leg in Tree pose.

2. Press your left foot into the wall.

3. Raise your arms above your head to the floor behind you.

4. Grasp your left wrist with your right hand.

5. Crab walk your upper body a little to the right.

6. Gently pull on your left wrist.

7. Repeat on the other side.

FALLEN TREE PRONE

1. Lie on your belly.

2. Press your left foot into the wall.

3. Bend your right leg and place it in Tree pose.

4. Place your elbows just in front of your shoulders and press up onto your forearms. If the low back or sacrum is not at ease, come back down to lie on the belly.

5. Repeat on the other side.

SEATED TREE

1. Come to a seated position.

2. Straighten your legs and press both of your feet into the wall.

3. Draw your right knee up so your right foot is in line with your left knee.

4. Press your left foot into the wall.

5. Turn your right knee out to the right.

6. Connect your right foot to thigh and left thigh to foot.

7. Bow over your left leg.

SUPPORTED TREE

1. Stand with your back to the wall.

2. Lift your right leg into Tree; hold for a few breaths before changing to the left side.

3. Press your back into the wall to feel supported.

4. Repeat on the other side.

WILLOW TREE

1. Turn to the long edge of the mat with your right hip facing the wall.

2. Stand one arm's length away from the wall.

3. Press your right hand into the wall like a foot.

4. Engage the arm by isometrically turning the palm to the right.

5. Lift your right knee into Tree pose.

6. Lift your left hand to the sky and bow to your right as if you were to touch the wall.

7. Repeat on the other side.

Forest Bathing

1 FLOWING TREE	**2** WILLOW SUPINE	**3** FALLEN TREE PRONE
4 SEATED TREE	**5** SUPPORTED TREE	**6** WILLOW TREE

Teaching Notes

+ The postures in Forest Bathing can be done without a wall.

+ See Ahimsa for further wall postures.

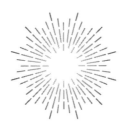

CHAPTER SIX

MEANINGFUL MIDDLES

This section dives deeper both into the physical body and the age-old philosophy of the wisdom traditions. Once the body is warmed up, the mind starts to clear, and we become more open to exploring this ancient art and science we call yoga.

This section pays tribute to the elements, the deities, the sutras, and the chakras as relatable themes in the yoga classroom and in your life. By honouring traditions and different forms of the practice we keep the yoga alive in a modern-day context.

The Five Elements—salutations

The Chakras—blueprint chakra poses

The Vayus—subtle energetic support for both the elements and the chakras

The Deities—flow, vinyasa

The Sutras—explore different styles of yoga

SALUTE THE ELEMENTS

When one tugs at a single thing in nature, one finds it attached to the rest of the world.

JOHN MUIR

We are a species, one of many species that make up part of our natural world. The elements or *bhuta*—earth, water, fire, air, and space—exist within us and outside of us. It is the quality and balance of them within that will lead us towards the fullest and healthiest expression of our life. Without them moving through us we are led towards decay.

Nature is in constant flux and we are part of that biorhythm. The earth moves inwards and cohesively contracts to bring all things together. Water flows downwards and eliminates what is not needed. Fire burns, sending everything it consumes upwards, and air moves outwards trying to enter anything that it touches. Ether is all-pervasive. Nature expands and contracts, moves upwards and downwards, gathers and disperses energy. This energy that flows through nature also flows through our bones, veins, lymph vessels, and pathways, and to keep in balance we must learn to harness and move it wisely throughout our bodies.

By understanding the movement of energy within us we are able to adjust, move, or enhance and direct flow—in balance this ensures the health of the mind and body.

Spiritually, the grace and wonder of the elements is beautifully told in the story of Krishna as a child.

Child Krishna Holds the Universe in his Mouth

One day Krishna and his friends were playing in their yard. Krishna, like many children, decided to taste the earth by placing it in his mouth. Krishna's friends ran to his mother to tell on him.

His mother, Yashoda Ma, scolded the boy for being mischievous and demanded he open his mouth.

When Yashoda peered in, she fell into wonderment. She saw within her tiny boy's mouth all of the Universe, plants and animals, the oceans, planets and stars and galaxies. She saw all of the elements and the width, breadth, and height of the world. She saw hope and loss, gain and shame, memories and desire, life and death. She saw his divinity, love, and the eternal essence of life.

Salute the Elements marries the intelligence of the elements to the grace of Salutations.

The *pancha maha bhuta*, or Ayurvedic five-element theory, says everything that exists—our constitution or *dosha*, the food we eat, the seasons—is a combination of

+ earth

+ water

+ fire

+ air or wind

+ space

When the elements combine, they form the **doshas**:

+ kapha: earth and water

+ pitta: water and fire

+ vata: air and space

Each of the elements has a **guiding principle:**

+ earth: the principle of inertia

+ water: the principle of cohesion

+ fire: the principle of radiance

+ wind: the principle of vibration

+ ether: the principle of pervasiveness

Each of the elements is associated with a **vayu:**

+ earth: apana

+ water: vyana

+ fire: samana

+ wind: prana

+ ether: udana

Each of the elements has a **quality**:

+ earth: grounding, stable, centred, present

+ water: flowing, able to change, adaptable, fluid, flexible, harmonising

+ fire: courage, stimulating, intense, expressive, drives us forwards

+ air: frees and liberates

+ space: the container for all the elements

Each of the elements guides a **specific chakra**:

+ earth: first chakra or muladhara

+ water: second chakra or svadhisthana

+ fire: third chakra or manipura

+ air: fourth chakra or anahata

+ space: fifth chakra or vishuddha

The elements relate to **different poses**:

+ earth: standing poses, work with the feet and legs, balance poses, foundational poses, grounding poses, focus on slow steady poses and movement, working with the lower body and building strength.

+ water: motion, graceful transitions, flowing movements, vinyasa, postures associated with the sacral area, hip openers, circular movements, ocean breath (Ujjayi).

+ fire: transformation, longer holds, challenging poses, expressive movement, core work, arm balances, upper body strengthening, bandha or energetic locks, meditation.

+ air: creating space in the shoulders and chest, backbends, finding expansiveness in the poses, pranayama practices.

+ space: creating or bringing attention to the space in our body, bringing attention to the container of our body, using sound and mantra practices, drishti practice.

Teaching Notes

+ Choose one element to work with for a week or month.

+ Work with an element to balance an excess in your constitution. If you are feeling lethargic (earth) opt for a fire practice to bring you into balance. If you feel ungrounded, choose a cooling earth practice to ground and stabilise you.

+ The elements move from gross (earth) to more subtle qualities (space). The yoga class can be themed using all of the elements in one class, starting from steady grounding poses (earth) and working your way to a yoga nidra (space).

+ Each element is associated with a chakra. See the section on Wheels.

+ Create an element meditation. Start with earth and move up through the elements bringing attention to where they are found and how they are manifested in your body.

+ Choose one element and a body part. Theme your class on the feet and legs and how this relates to the qualities of earth.

+ Investigate bhuta (element), shuddi (purification) meditation, a tantric practice to purify the elements within.

+ Bring the qualities of the elements into your salutations. See below in Salute the Elements.

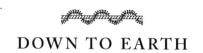

DOWN TO EARTH

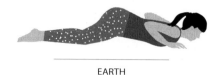

EARTH

The miracle is to walk on the green earth,
dwelling deeply in the present moment and feeling truly alive.

THICH NHAT HANH

To the Mind

Prithvi/bhumi:	element of earth/soil
Sense organ:	nose and smell
Chakra:	muladhara
Direction:	north
Complementary oils:	plant roots—jatamansi, angelica root, patchouli, valerian root, or Indian spikehead, thought to be the oil Mary Magdalene rubbed on the feet of Jesus before the last supper
Essential vocabulary:	patient, grounded, centring, fertile, warm, comfort, reliable, abundant, stability, stable, connection, safety, mula
Mula:	root. Mula bandha is a contraction of the toilet muscles to contain energy in the body.
Imbalance:	shows up as worry, a knot of uneasiness in the stomach, overthinking

QUALITIES OF EARTH

- foundational
- gives structure
- dependable
- provider and nurturer

To the Heart

Our human form is a construct of the element earth—skin and bones, muscles and hair, blood, cells, and tissues.

We arose from one source, and we return to this source. Our passage here on Earth will walk us hundreds of thousands of miles through an infinite timeline and complex ecosystem. So often we are wanderers, sleepwalking the earth, searching for safety, stability, love. We may walk in fear, loneliness, and confusion, forgetting where we live.

Thich Nhat Hanh, in his walking meditation 'I have arrived, I am home,' encourages us in every step to remember our faithful address in the present moment. When you are tired of running away, when you are homesick or feel peace has left you, come back to your safe haven with the pulse of walking meditation.

To the Body

❧ *Down to Earth* ☙

In Down to Earth we pay homage to gentle grounding opening poses and an earthy, ground dwelling salutation.

BHUMISPARSHA MUDRA—EARTH BEARS WITNESS MUDRA

One of the iconic stories of Buddhism tells of when the Buddha became enlightened.

After many days and nights of roaming, the Buddha sat under the Bodhi tree and vowed to stay there until he became enlightened. Just before his enlightenment, the demonic celestial king, Mara, appeared as the representation of the Buddha's shadow side. Mara taunted the Buddha, trying to distract him and throw him off his path. Enraged at Buddha's successful enlightenment, he called out to him 'Who do you think you are?' He demanded the Buddha should prove that he had been awakened. The Buddha touched the ground with his right hand, and the earth called out 'I am your witness,' upon which the morning star appeared in the sky to mark the supreme moment of enlightenment.

SEATED BHUMISPARSHA MUDRA

1. Place the left hand open on the left thigh. This is the beginning of Dhyana (meditation) mudra.
2. Place the five fingers of the right hand to touch the ground with an open palm.

What do you want to call up? What do you want the earth to bear witness to today? What would you like to summon into your life or hold accountable in your heart? As you place your hand on the earth, feel the resonance of that commitment move into you and take shape and form as an intention.

RECLINED BUTTERFLY

1. Lie on your back.
2. Bring the soles of your feet together.
3. Let your knees fall out wide.

WINDSHIELD WIPERS

1. Lie on your back.
2. Take your feet to the edges of your mat.
3. Let your knees fall to the right.
4. Repeat on the other side.

RECLINED FIGURE FOUR

1. Lie on your back.
2. Bend your knees.
3. Place your left ankle on your right knee.

4. Lift your right leg.
5. Thread your hands through the keyhole in your legs and hold the back of the right thigh or shin.

RECLINED FIGURE FOUR TWIST

1. From Reclined Figure Four, drop your left foot to the floor outside of your right thigh.
2. Keep your left knee facing the ceiling.

RECLINED EAGLE TWIST

1. From Reclined Figure Four Twist, slip your left knee farther around your right thigh, creating Eagle Legs.
2. Repeat from Windshield Wipers to Eagle Twist on the other side.

Earth

| 1 RECLINED BUTTERFLY | 2 WINDSHIELD WIPERS | 3 RECLINED FIGURE FOUR |

| 4 RECLINED FIGURE FOUR TWIST | 5 EAGLE TWIST |

❧ *Earth Salutation* ☙

1. Sit in Thunderbolt.
2. Inhale, reach arms overhead.
3. Exhale, fold into Child's pose.
4. Inhale, move into Tabletop.
5. Exhale, lower your chest between your hands.

6. Inhale, move into Cobra pose.
7. Exhale, full Pranam. *I bow to the earth.*
8. Inhale, Cobra pose.
9. Exhale, Child's pose.
10. Inhale, Thunderbolt.

-------- *Earth Salutation* --------

Teaching Notes

+ Keep poses low to the ground. Emphasis on creating steadiness, stability, and strength emulates the characteristics of the earth.

+ Explore Squat pose, which drops and softens the pelvis.

+ Bringing energy downwards within the body calms and centres the mind. Exploration of apana vayu, (downwards-moving energy) will cultivate this, as will standing strong into your feet and legs. Warrior poses drive our feet and weight into the earth.

+ Work with the feet. Foot massage, feet and ankle circles, rolling a ball under the feet, and Toe Squat remind students of their foundations and connection to the earth.

+ Poses on hands and knees not only bring students physically closer to the earth but embody the crawling and exploration stage of development where children eat dirt to explore their world. (See also Krishna Holds the Universe in His Mouth.)

+ Any poses that invoke the muladhara chakra work with the earth element.

+ Full prostration, or Pranam, is a deep and trusting pose that calls us to surrender to the will of something higher than ourselves. Insert this pose between salutations or sets of poses.

+ Balancing poses remind us to adjust and connect when feeling unstable. Explore Tree, Warrior Three, or Standing Knee to Chest.

+ Mula bandha, or root lock, and poses that call attention to the sacrum, pelvis, and tailbone work the earth element. The tailbone is like an ancestral root, drawing us into the earth.

+ Students that have excess 'air' and 'space' and who seem fractured or distracted will be balanced through the earth element practices. When we are restless and vigilant, we move away from the centre or the grounded aspects of our being. Invite students to note how they feel before the practice and how they feel after.

+ Prithvi mudra connects the thumb with the ring finger (earth finger). Prithvi means 'the vast one' and is also the name for the earth.

To Your Life

Throughout history, the ground was our home—we slept, cooked, and lived in close connection to the earth. In modern society, as we have become more disconnected with our environment; our bodies hardly come into contact with the sweet soil.

The therapeutic benefits of grounding, or earthing, are still being understood. It is believed that by touching our feet, hands, or body to the earth, we assimilate her healing, anti-inflammatory energy (electrons). Gardening, walking barefoot, and swimming are some ways we can practice returning to our roots.

+ Spend thirty minutes walking barefoot or putting your hands into the soil, tasting its nourishment with all your senses.

+ Walking meditations create reciprocity with our bodies and the earth. As you walk, feel the sponginess of the feet, the balance required, the actions of the toes, the rebounding of the earth. Walk as Thich Nhat Hanh says: 'as if your feet were kissing the earth.'

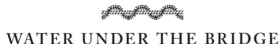

WATER UNDER THE BRIDGE

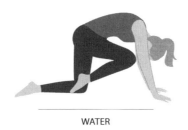

WATER

You are not a drop in the ocean. You are the entire ocean, in a drop.

RUMI

To the Mind

Jala: element of water

Sense organ: tongue, the sense of taste

Chakra: svadhisthana, the second chakra, associated with creativity and sensuality

Direction: west

Complementary oils: extracts from stems and trunks, sandalwood, cedarwood, ginger, jasmine, and clary sage

Essential vocabulary: flow, create, receive, receptivity, fluid, hydrate, nourish, not stagnate, moist, cool, tides and tidal, cohesion, soothing, softens, adhere

Imbalance: shows up as lack of creativity, addictions, emotional outbursts, reproductive, kidney, and bladder issues

QUALITIES OF WATER

- Water cleanses. As water passes through its channels, it takes out the old and makes way for the new.
- Water reflects. In still water we can see our reflection.
- Water is dynamic and flows. We must flow through our life to avoid stagnation.

- Water nourishes and lubricates. Without water, we dry and perish.
- Water unifies. We are one drop in the ocean of life. Remember you are a part of the whole. Power is gained from collaboration and support from the collective whole.
- Water is flexible: it takes the shape of its container. For us to grow and evolve, we must learn to mould with what life is presenting.
- Water is patient and persistent: it finds the path of least resistance.
- Water stays true: water to ice, ice to water; it comes back to its true self.

Beneath the earthiness of the skin and bones lies the cohesive, fluid body. Composed of blood, plasma, cerebral spinal fluid, synovial fluid, cellular fluid, and interstitial fluid, it makes up around 70 percent of our composition.

This watery body hydrates and nourishes us, dissolving and carrying nutrients to our cells and flushing out unwanted by-products. It protects the pathways in which it flows: brain, mouth, throat, stomach, joints, and reproductive organs.

This saline conduit of life runs through the tributaries, or *nadis*, of our body. As the waters flow, they touch nearly every organ and every cell, communicating with and connecting our internal pathways. It is said our fluid body has a similar constitution to the sea, and in our mother's womb we were quite literally floating in this sea of life.

To the Heart

GO WITH THE FLOW

As water dances through our limbs, as it flows, moves, and morphs, it reminds us that flow is our natural state. Moving the body in rhythm, going with the flow, and learning to let go are ways to honour the water element within. We always have a choice. To swim against the tide, to cling on to the bank, or to float in synchronicity with our life. When we become like Teflon, nothing sticks, and we do not get stuck.

To go with the flow of your life means to accept your life as it is unfolding. It doesn't mean that we don't have daily annoyances and situations that we resist; it's just that we become better at identifying the places that are gritty and stuck. If we examine these places with curiosity, we may find a teaching or a gift.

Is it possible that the places you are most stuck are the places where you have the most valuable lessons?

Is it possible that where you don't want to flow, is where you need to?

Some days your life will seem like a riptide, where you are dragged up and down through choppy waters. On other days it will be a gentle eddy on a clear blue day where you float seamlessly through life.

Be open to them all.

Go with the flow.

To the Body

❧ *Water Under the Bridge* ☙

These beginning movements are variations on Bridge pose and are a metaphor for the flowing, connecting nature of water. The Salutation continues the theme with a water mandala flow.

UJJAYI

Ud: upward or superior in rank

Jaya: conquest, victory, triumph

Ujjayi: victorious; sometimes called Conqueror's breath. The tidal estuary of the breath moves in and out. It is a high, bold king tide or sometimes so low and quiet it almost disappears. Ujjayi breath is the perfect complement for the water element, with its soothing tidal hum.

Ujjayi breath is the sound of the ocean and deep-sea diving.
It is the hollow whisper of a shell held to an ear and warm breath on a cold mirror.
It is a slant of sun that pierces your lungs with life and pours energy into your soul.

KEY POINTS

+ It has a sound. (The sound of Ujjayi is made by blocking off the glottis and breathing through a restricted windpipe, creating a sound like the ocean.) The sound, however, doesn't need to be loud, just audible to yourself.

+ Both the inhale and exhale should be smooth and even.

UJJAYI SCRIPT

Sit like lightning, in Thunderbolt. Feel the diamond-like qualities of determination, strength, and indestructibility to face what needs to be faced.

Today we will practise Ujjayi breathing. Ujjayi means victorious; we practice in order to conquer ourselves.

Breathe through your nose but feel like you are breathing through a straw in the base of your throat. Feel the constriction in the back of the throat. Listen to the sound that arises.

In and out.

Keep a steady tempo, just you and your breath.
Notice the oceanic sound that you make; trace the sound deep into your being.
Until your breath becomes the ocean itself.

Keep breathing in and out as if you were drawing a fine silk thread through the eye of a needle.

Water

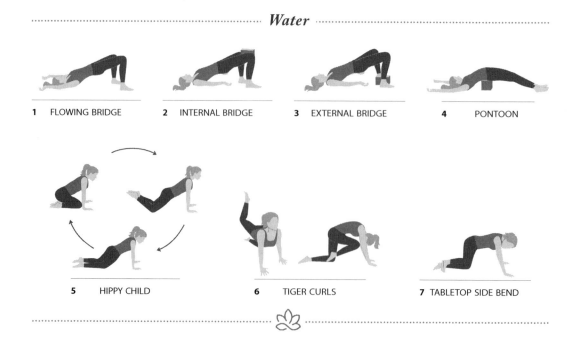

1   FLOWING BRIDGE   2   INTERNAL BRIDGE   3   EXTERNAL BRIDGE   4   PONTOON

5   HIPPY CHILD   6   TIGER CURLS   7   TABLETOP SIDE BEND

FLOWING BRIDGE

Creating a breath rhythm in Flowing Bridge:

1. Lie on your back with your hands by your sides and your knees bent, feet on the floor.
2. Inhale, lift your hips and your arms until your fingers touch the floor behind your head.
3. Exhale, drop your hips and arms down by your sides.
4. Roll in and out of your Bridge like a wave.

INTERNAL BRIDGE

This pose strengthens the internal rotators of the hips.

1. Lie in Constructive Rest pose with your knees together and your legs bent.
2. Place a block between your knees and squeeze the block.
3. Your feet will be slightly wider than your knees.
4. Place your hands on your belly.
5. Inhale, lift your hips and arms as in Flowing Bridge.
6. Exhale, lower your hips to the floor.
7. Repeat five times.

EXTERNAL BRIDGE

This pose strengthens the external rotators of the hips.

1. Lie on your back and place a block between your feet.
2. Your knees will be slightly wider than your feet.

3. Squeeze the block between your feet.
4. Inhale, lift your hips into Bridge pose and your arms up over your head as in flowing Bridge.
5. Exhale, drop your arms by your sides as you lower your pelvis to the floor.
6. Repeat five times.

PONTOON

1. Place a block under your sacrum.
2. Stretch your arms out above you onto the floor.
3. Stretch your legs forwards.

HIPPY CHILD

1. Start with your seat on your heels.
2. Move the chest forwards, so your shoulders are over your wrists.
3. Circle your hips to the right in clockwise rotations.
4. Repeat in an anticlockwise direction.

TIGER CURLS

1. From Tabletop, inhale and stretch your left leg out behind you.
2. Exhale, curl your knee to your nose.
3. Repeat on the other side.

TABLETOP SIDE BEND

1. From Tabletop, arch your spine to look at your right hip.
2. Arch your spine to look at your left hip.
3. Move back and forth between the sides.

☞ *Water Salutation* ☜

The Water Salutation below is a mandala—a circle with a centre. Flowing between sides and back to front, the body becomes a fluid circle of movement. You can add any poses to the mandala. The trick in teaching one is to lead with the right leg twice, then the left leg twice, which will take you in a complete circle.

SALUTATION

1. Start in Mountain.
2. Inhale, reach your arms skyward.
3. Exhale, hinge at your hips and bow to the floor.
4. Inhale, lift your shoulders in line with your hips.
5. Exhale, step back to Down Dog.
6. Inhale, come into High Plank.
7. Exhale, lower your body to the ground.
8. Inhale, arch your spine into Cobra.
9. Exhale, Down Dog.

MANDALA BEGINS

1. Inhale, your right leg into the sky.
2. Exhale, step your right leg through to your right hand.
3. Inhale, Crescent Warrior.
4. Exhale, Warrior Two.
5. Inhale, Star pose.
6. Exhale, Warrior Two, facing the back of the room.
7. Inhale, spin on your back foot, lift your heel, and turn your chest to Crescent Warrior.
8. Vinyasa (High Plank, Low Plank, Cobra or Up Dog, Down Dog).

Repeat three more times.

On the second round, lift the right leg again.

On the third round, lead with the left leg.

On the fourth round, lead with the left leg.

You will complete a circle.

Water Salutation

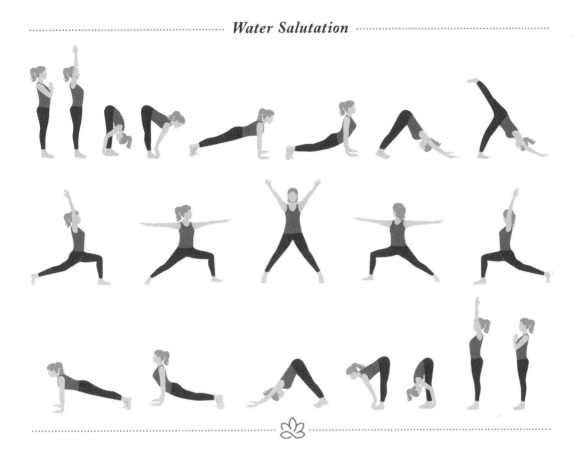

Teaching Notes

✦ Opt for flowing repetitions of poses and or sequences. Poses such as Tiger Curls, Half Lift, and Cobra can be repeated in flowing sets of three.

✦ Ladder Technique

The ladder technique is a good way to incorporate flow and rhythm into classes. Choose a pose and add a new pose each cycle or flow.

Using Warrior One as an example,

· Round 1—Warrior One
· Round 2—Warrior One, add Warrior Two
· Round 3—Warrior One and Warrior Two, add Reverse Warrior
· Round 4—Warrior One, Two, and Reverse, add Side Plank, and so on.

✦ Water is soft and fluid but has a power to it when needed—riptides, tidal waves, flooded rivers—that can move anything in its way. Play with this duality in finding strength but fluidity in poses.

✦ Work with the low belly, the pelvis, and the two pelvic halves to honour water's attachment to the second chakra. Flowing in and out of Pigeon creates fluidity while working and softening the connection of the hip/pelvic region.

✦ Creativity is a by-product of the water element being in balance. As an alternative to the Mandala Salutation, consider putting on some music and letting students flow organically.

✦ Attention to transitions between poses is a crucial way to maintain fluidity and playfulness in your practice. Move smoothly and creatively between postures without jarring.

✦ Water practice and flows complement full moon–inspired classes.

✦ Boat pose and its variations play with the water theme.

✦ Supported Legs up the Wall helps students feel and visualise the draining of fluid/lymph from the feet into the watery bowl of the pelvis.

✦ As much as water flows, it can also be still, dark, and deep. Finishing a class with one long-held yin pose such as Pontoon contrasts the flowing movements while appreciating the yin-like quality of water.

To Your Life

The wave does not need to die to become water, she already is water.

THICH NHAT HANH

Tidal water takes away what is not needed on the outgoing tide and refreshes on the incoming. What old ideas or ways of being would you like to flush out?

Being stuck in any way, be it an idea, a habit, or a relationship, will bring disharmony to the heart, mind, and body, and create stagnation. Are there any areas of your life where you feel stuck? Maybe in a job or relationship, there may be a feeling of stagnation. What would it take to hydrate these places?

Do you consider yourself flexible?

Are you willing to take on what life is presenting you rather than pushing it away? Resilience is a strength. Only hard, brittle branches break; soft and supple ones sway and bend.

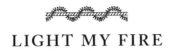

LIGHT MY FIRE

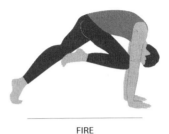

FIRE

Set your life on fire, seek those who fan your flames.
RUMI

To the Mind

Agni: element of fire

Sense organ: sight. When this element is in balance, our perception is sharp, and our inner luminosity glows through our eyes.

Chakra: manipura

Direction: south

Complementary oils: flower and spice oils, clove, cardamom, lavender, rosemary

Essential vocabulary: insight, strength, courage, healing, discernment, purifies both matter and energy, ember, glow, burn through, transform, passion, burn out, burn the candle at both ends, combustion, passion

Imbalance: shows up as overconfidence, arrogance, bossiness, intensity, burn out, inability to focus, digestive issues

QUALITIES OF FIRE

- Fire is about discernment.
- To be able to sort the wheat from the chaff, to know what is right or wrong, to be able to detect the truth, and the possession of a sharp intellect, are signs of balanced fire within. When the element is imbalanced, the mind can become dull and stuck.
- Fire has the potential to be destructive.

- But in the destruction new life is born. Just as controlled fires burn off the old debris in a forest to make way for the new, fire in our life can transform and evolve us by razing what is no longer needed to make space for new ideas, new ways of being.
- Fire generates energy for the body, just as the sun generates it for the earth.
- Fire encourages us to live to the fullest, encouraging joy, love, and compassion in our lives.
- 'To raise' means to lift up or elevate; 'to raze' is to burn down and destroy. Fire has both of these powers, to lift us up or to burn us out.
- Fire liberates energy from its source. Consider where you need to put your energy today. How much energy do you truly have for what it is you need to do? Do you tend to 'overdo' things and scatter your energy in many different directions? Like a magnifying glass in the sun held over paper, try a more focussed approach to one task today.

To the Heart

You are the emissary of your core values, the messenger of what you hold true.

You have the power within to stand up for what you believe in, and for the things in life you value.

Sometimes strength means to stay and be still, while at other times it means to fight—for what you believe in, for your values, for others, for your legacy.

At the centre of your being is your personal sun, a radiance that never dies.

We all have within us intensity of heat, perseverance, commitment, discipline; an inner fire that we can call upon any time.

Feel the fire inside igniting you like the lamps of a lighthouse, calling you to walk through your challenges and adversities. The heat will create ash from your old stories and soften the edges of everything sharp.

All your fires are your teachers.

And all your lessons hold the seed of radical transformation.

To the Body

⟩ *Fire* ⟨

In fire we bring heat and strength to the core muscles, both in the opening sequence and during the Salutation. Kapalabhati and an Agni meditation will bring an added flourish to this fiery practice.

KAPALABHATI

Kapala: skull

Bhati: shine or clean

Kapalabhati: skull shining breath. After practising it you may feel a lightness or electricity in the skull. The breath is said to clean our mind and our perceptions, cleanse the respiratory system, improve circulation, and strengthen and tone the abdominal muscles.

KEY POINTS

+ The vigour of the exhale is more important than the speed.
+ Control the abdominal walls—this is where all movement comes from.
+ Push the breath out with your lower belly.
+ The breath is performed with short sharp exhales through both nostrils.
+ Feel the belly snap back like a staccato note on each exhale.
+ The in-breath comes of its own accord, arising from the vacuum of the lungs.
+ Keep the head, neck, and shoulders still.
+ Keep your nostrils soft.
+ If you feel dizzy, return to normal breathing.

KAPALABHATI SCRIPT

Cradle your palms on your hip bones and low belly and cough.

These are the muscles you use in Kapalabhati.

Begin with a long slow inhale and exhale. Feel yourself settling here.

Inhale to the top of the lungs.

Exhale completely.

Inhale to around 70 percent of your capacity.

Exhale powerfully through both nostrils from the pit of your belly.

Like a steam train starting off, start slowly; breathe as a community.

Listen to the person next to you, synchronise with them.

When we breathe together, we recognise our connection.

At the end of the fifteenth exhale, finish completely right to the tail end.

Take a generous breath in, as deep as possible, drop your chin to your chest, and energetically lift the front of your throat, like an elegant swan's neck.

Stay here and relax into the fullness, as if the breath was holding you.

Find your edge; shift from thinking to feeling.

When you are ready, lift the chin, let go of the breath, stay still and feel.

AGNI MEDITATION

This could also be done with a candle flame and eyes open.

Sit in a comfortable position. Allow the curves of your spine to be present.

When we hold a magnifying glass to paper and allow the heat of the sun to concentrate on one spot, that spot intensifies.

Close your eyes and imagine a flame, fire, or bonfire of your choosing. Put all your attention behind the flames. See their shape and colour. Feel their heat.

Now call to mind something that you would like to ignite or burn through in your life.

We now offer this up to Agni[7], the god of fire.

We call upon you, Agni, to light our path, to guide our way, to ignite the fire that dwells within each and every one of us.

Through your power may we process and digest the things we have swallowed whole and looked away from.

May we burn through and clear some of our most tightly held secrets, beliefs, and hidden commands that run our life, so nothing stands in the way of our evolution.

May we process, digest, transform, assimilate, and ultimately free ourselves.

---

[7] The *Rig Veda* (sacred truth), is one of the oldest and most important Hindu texts dedicated to various gods in the form of hymns. The first words are dedicated to Agni, the fire god, celebrating his importance as both an element and a deity. *'Oh Agni I adore you.'*

BELLY BREATHING

1. Lie on your back.
2. Place your hands on your belly.
3. Begin to take long slow breaths into the centre of your being as if you were trying to fill yourself up.
4. Feel softness and movement under your hands.

SINGLE LEG LOWERS

1. Lie on your back.
2. Hug your right knee into your chest.
3. Lift your left leg to the sky.
4. Exhale, lower your left leg to a few centimetres off the ground.
5. Inhale, lift your left leg back to the sky.
6. Repeat this movement five to ten times.
7. Repeat on the other side.

SCISSOR LEGS

1. Lie on your back.
2. Inhale, lift your legs into the air with your feet facing the ceiling.
3. Exhale, drop your right leg down so it hovers off the floor. Exhale, cross it to the left.
4. At the same time, move your left leg to the right to create 'scissor' legs.
5. Inhale, lift both legs back to the starting position with your feet facing the ceiling.
6. Repeat on the other side.

TWISTY CORE

1. Lie on your back and bring your legs to Tabletop.
2. Seal your inner knees and inner ankles together.
3. Place your arms into 'cactus' arms and pin your shoulders down to the mat.
4. Inhale, drop your knees to the right 45 degrees.
5. Exhale, use your core to bring them back to centre.
6. Inhale, drop your knees to the left 45 degrees.
7. Exhale, use your core to bring them back to centre.
8. Finish with a gentle twist to both sides.

BIRD DOG

1. Come to Tabletop posture on your hands and knees.
2. Firm your low ribs into your spine.
3. Inhale, stretch your right arm out to the wall in front of you.
4. Stretch your left leg out to the wall behind you.
5. Stay here for three breaths.
6. Repeat on the other side.

Fire

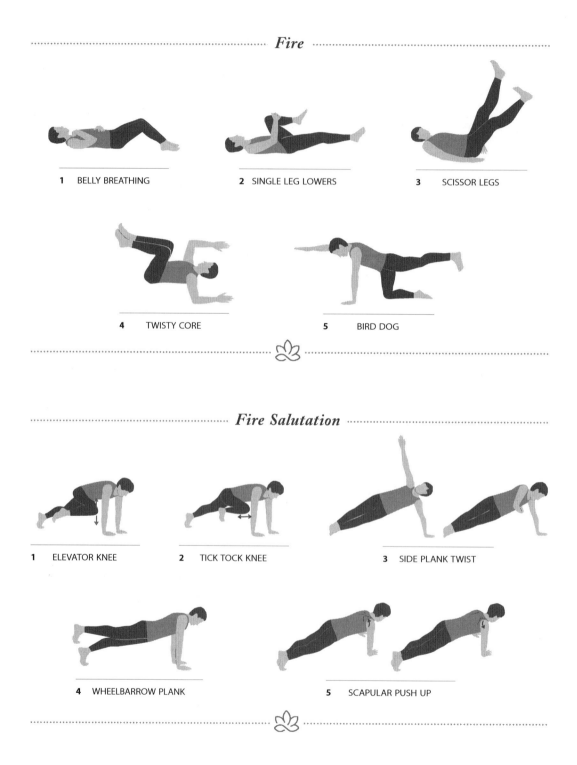

1 BELLY BREATHING

2 SINGLE LEG LOWERS

3 SCISSOR LEGS

4 TWISTY CORE

5 BIRD DOG

Fire Salutation

1 ELEVATOR KNEE

2 TICK TOCK KNEE

3 SIDE PLANK TWIST

4 WHEELBARROW PLANK

5 SCAPULAR PUSH UP

❧ *Fire Salutation* ☙

Adding heat to a Sun Salutation through core work ignites the physical heat in the body. Having the power to stay and burn through difficult situations is life training for off the mat.

Add any of these Plank/core variations into your favourite salutation as a substitute for Chaturanga or Low Plank.

ELEVATOR KNEE

1. Come into High Plank.
2. Bring your right knee towards your right armpit.
3. Inhale, drop your right knee towards your right wrist.
4. Exhale, lift your right knee towards your right armpit.
5. Repeat this up-and-down movement with your knee three times.

TICK TOCK KNEE

1. Come into High Plank.
2. Bring your right knee towards your right elbow.
3. Swing your right knee towards your left elbow.
4. Go back and forth with your knee like a pendulum on a clock for around ten swings.

SIDE PLANK TWIST

1. Come into Side Plank on your right side.
2. Inhale, open your left hand to the sky.
3. Exhale, curl your left hand under your right ribs.
4. Repeat three times.

WHEELBARROW PLANK

1. Come into High Plank and firm your belly.
2. Inhale, lift your right foot ten centimetres off the ground.
3. Exhale, place your right foot on the ground.
4. Repeat on the left side.
5. Alternate right and left for four sets.

SCAPULAR PUSH UP

1. From High Plank, drop your knees to the floor or stay on your toes.
2. Inhale, drop your chest between your shoulder blades, keep your arms straight.
3. Exhale, press into the floor and round your upper back to the sky.

Teaching Notes

+ Choose poses that build heat, especially around the core. However, in the heat of summer or the heat of the day you may prefer to take a 'cooling' approach to balance the heat.

+ Strength poses such as Plank and her variations remind us to step up to the power within.

+ Fire is the primary element of digestion. Not just of our food but also our thoughts and what we take in through our senses. When we don't digest something, it builds up and becomes a nagging pain in the mind, heart, or body. Twists stimulate the digestive organs, e.g., Lunge Twist, Twisted Half Moon, seated twists.

+ Hold standing poses a little longer to build heat, e.g. Chair, Warriors.

+ Our feet can help us change course quickly if we are not on the right path. They can speed us up, slow us down, or move us in the direction of our goals and desires. Target the feet, as they are the physical representations of fire in our body.

+ Flowing vinyasa style will build heat, especially when intermingled with core strength actions.

+ Fire requires air to keep it burning. Choose stronger breath techniques such as Kapalabhati, Bhastrika (Bellows breath), or Agni Sara (fire essence) for more active classes, and cooling steady breath such as Sitali for slower classes.

+ With yin or restorative classes, opt for poses that stimulate the belly, such as Supine Twist, Deer Twist, or Child's pose. The story of Icarus is a metaphor for finding the right amount of effort in yin or restorative classes. Icarus, while trying to escape his labyrinth prison, flew too close to the sun, melting his feather and wax wings.

+ Agni Stambasana, or Fire Log pose, is a physical metaphor for the element of fire. It is also very heating for the hips. The shape of the pose is said to arise from the funeral pyres at the Ganges. The placement of the shins represents the triangular stack of wood used for cremation.

+ Kali flow incorporates fire and the energy of transformation.

To Your Life

What is your relationship to adversity? *Carrot, Egg, Coffee Beans*, is a simple story to illustrate how each of us can differ in times of hardship. Life requires us to walk through the adversities and challenges it presents.

We each have a choice—to sidestep, battle, or transform.

CARROT, EGG, COFFEE BEANS

A young woman, after suffering some setbacks, asked her grandmother about how to cope with adversity.

The grandmother put three pots of water on to boil on the campfire and placed in them a carrot, an egg, and some coffee beans.

After some time, she turned off the heat and asked her granddaughter what she saw.

The carrot started out strong and hard but had turned to mush.

The egg had become hard and impenetrable, losing its softness.

The coffee granules transmuted into coffee.

The grandmother explained that each of these things had faced the same adversity in the form of heat, but they reacted differently.

One collapsed, one put up its shields, and the other transformed itself.

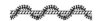

A BREATH OF FRESH AIR

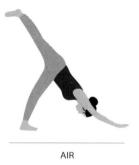

AIR

The wind blows wherever it pleases.

JOHN 3.8

To the Mind

Vayu: element of air. *Pneuma* is the Greek word for air in motion, which also means the vital force or spirit of a person

Sense organ: touch and skin

Chakra: anahata

Direction: east

Complementary oils: leaves from plants, tulsi, peppermint, eucalyptus, tea tree, the oils that help you breathe

Essential vocabulary: learning, knowledge, the mind and intellect, curiosity, imagination, ideas, wisdom, billowy, flowing, mobile, agile, dynamic, moving, uplifting

Imbalance: shows up as agitation, feeling ungrounded, restlessness, and racing thoughts

QUALITIES OF AIR

Her qualities are synonymous with the wind:

- movement, mobility, flowing
- lightness, clear, dry
- expansion

To the Heart

As ether starts to take visible form in the world, she appears as air. Her movement seeps and infuses into our bodies through our breath and swirls within our energetic pathways. She is carried in the tumbling leaves and the bustling clouds. Her breath is the voice of our soul.

Vayu represents all movement in the body. From the beating heart to the workings of the digestive system, from our coursing blood to the articulation of bones and joints. Vayu feeds and circulates energy freely while overseeing our nervous system. Too much air in the body can create an overexcited temperament, diarrhoea, and hypermobility, whereas too little is displayed as an overall sluggishness in the circulatory system.

Our thoughts, ideas, emotions, and creativity are carried on the currents of the air element.

Air is related to skin, the hands, and touch. Like a breath of air that knows no boundaries, we are able to touch others with love and we are open to receiving it when this element is in balance.

Air is the spontaneous force behind our life and dwindles as we look towards our later years, retirement, and lightening our load. Without her energy there is no life.

To the Body

❧ *Air* ☙

In Air we start with movements to release trapped air from the body and float into a dreamy, flowing Salutation.

OPENING CONTEMPLATION

Wind carries with it the power of creation in the floating seeds and the breath of new life. How can you harness this element into your life? How do you want to step into the flow of what the wind is calling you to do?

What would you like to breathe into creation?

BEGINNING BREATH— KUMBHAKA

Kumbha: container. The kumbha is also representative of the womb and its generative powers.

Kumbhaka is the practice of breath retention and is said to help store and conserve energy. As you practice, envisage energy entering your body and filling your body container.

The hold on the inhale builds heat and energy around the chest and solar plexus.

The hold on the exhale brings energy and vibration to the area below the navel and pelvic floor and is said to have a detoxifying effect.

REMINDERS

- Check there is no gripping, especially at the base of the throat.
- Keep the upper palate soft and spacious.
- If at any time it feels uncomfortable, let go of the technique and return to normal breathing.

KUMBHAKA SCRIPT

Sit comfortably.

Take a few long slow breaths and imagine you are saturating your lungs with beautiful life-sustaining energy.

Envisage your lungs as three-dimensional. When you inhale, fill them from the bottom to the top and from the centre outwards to the sides.

Now let's introduce kumbhaka, a pause.

At the top of your next inhale, pause the breath for a few counts.

When you are ready, let your breath out in a long stream through both nostrils.

Inhale, take the breath to a point between the eyes.

During the hold, fill this spot with light and let it spread out from your eyebrow centre.

See it flood behind the eyes and fill your entire skull.

Long, slow exhale.

Be intentional with your breath; direct it where it needs to go in your body.

You can continue to work with the eyebrow centre as your focus, but if there is another part of you that needs more love, more attention, take your breath there on the retention.

Continue with kumbhaka for a few more rounds of breath.

Each inhale brings in new life force, creativity.

Each exhale washes away the blocks in the way to your vision.

Sit here in contemplation for the next few minutes.

HALF WIND RELIEF

1. Lie on your back.
2. Squeeze your right knee into your chest.
3. Hold your right knee and make slow circles with your knee in both directions.

ANKLE CIRCLES

1. Bend your left leg and place your foot on the floor.
2. Cross your right ankle over your left thigh.
3. Circle your right ankle in both directions.
4. Repeat both moves on the other side.

WRIST CIRCLES

1. Sit comfortably.
2. Make a fist with your right hand.
3. Circle your wrist in both directions.
4. Repeat with your left hand.

SUFI CIRCLES

1. Place both hands on your thighs.
2. Circle your entire spine down towards your right knee, across your body, around to your left and back.
3. Circle in both directions.

.... *Air* ....

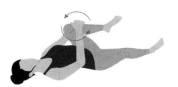

1 HALF WIND RELIEF

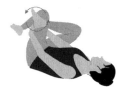

2 ANKLE CIRCLES

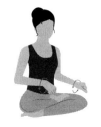

3 WRIST CIRCLES

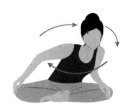

4 SUFI CIRCLES

❧ *Air Salutation* ❦

This salute works with the energy of flowing air.

Like a metronome, can you move consistently with the beat of the breath? The breath starts before the movement and continues right to the end of the movement.

Teaching note: count the breath for the students as below for a count of four or five; keep the beat consistent.

Remind students to not cheat themselves of full inhales but more importantly to release full exhales. When we don't fully exhale, we can't then take a full breath in.

DOWN DOG, HIGH PLANK

1. Begin in Downward Facing Dog.
2. Inhale, ripple forwards, bring your shoulders over your wrists.
3. Exhale, lift your hips up and away to Down Dog.
4. Repeat three times.

DOWN DOG, LAZY UP DOG

1. Inhale, ripple forwards, bring your shoulders over your wrists and drop your belly towards the floor. Keep your toes tucked.
2. Exhale, lift up and back to Down Dog.
3. Repeat three times.

DOWN DOG SPLIT, KNEE TO NOSE

1. Inhale, lift your right leg into the air.
2. Exhale, bring your shoulders over your wrists as you bring your right knee to your chest.
3. Repeat three times.
4. On the third Knee to Nose, step your right foot by your right hand.

5. Exhale, step your left foot to meet your right.
6. Fold.
7. Stand.
8. Fold.
9. Repeat on the left side.

QUARTER SUN SALUTATIONS

1. Stand in Mountain Pose.
2. Inhale, reach your arms overhead, 2, 3, 4.
3. Exhale, bring your hands to your heart, 2, 3, 4.
4. Repeat three times.

HALF SUN SALUTATIONS

1. Inhale, reach your arms overhead, 2, 3, 4.
2. Exhale, bow to the earth, 2, 3, 4.
3. Inhale, lift your heart up halfway, 2, 3, 4.
4. Exhale, Forward Fold, 2, 3, 4.
5. Inhale, lift your hips, chest, shoulders, and arms to the sky, 2, 3, 4.
6. Exhale, bring your hands to your heart, 2, 3, 4.
7. Repeat three times.

Air Salutation

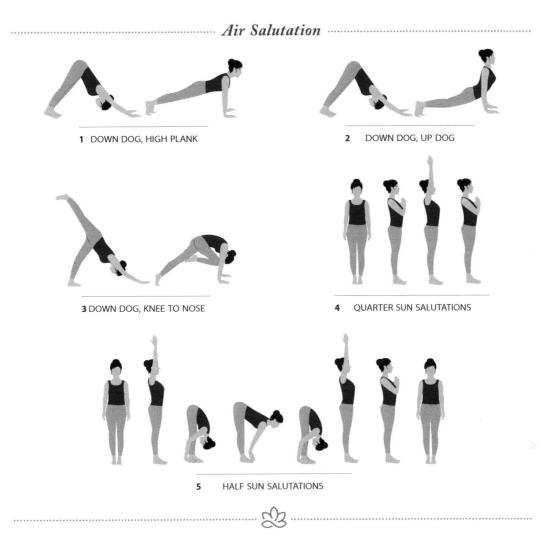

1 DOWN DOG, HIGH PLANK

2 DOWN DOG, UP DOG

3 DOWN DOG, KNEE TO NOSE

4 QUARTER SUN SALUTATIONS

5 HALF SUN SALUTATIONS

Teaching Notes

✦ The element of air is best balanced by slow, rhythmic movements, free flowing without obstruction.

✦ Routine is important, so consider repeating flows or predictable patterns of movement.

✦ Longer holds in poses provide a consistency that air needs to ground itself.

✦ Air is the element of anahata chakra. Poses that support anahata, such as heart opening poses that open the body from the back and front of the heart, embody the air element.

+ Air is responsible for all movement in the body. Poses that encourage movement of the circulatory system, such as vinyasa, or of the lymphatic system, such as inversions, encourage the flow of air throughout our interior.

+ Wind Relieving pose and its Pawanmuktasana series are excellent for removing stuck air in the joints.

+ Circling movements of the arms in Triangle, Warrior Two, and Side Angle continue to build on the theme of moving, circulating patterns of air.

+ The air element stimulates creativity. Consider putting on some inspiring music and moving like no one is watching. Creative entries and exits from poses, creative salutations, and creative versions of poses are ways we can play with air.

+ Notice how the wind changes during the day. Sometimes it is strong and forceful, at other times a whisper. Does the wind affect your moods? If we are predominantly vata (air and ether) in constitution (according to Ayurveda), we might find ourselves thrown off balance with strong winds and constant movement. Grounding earth poses balance an out-of-kilter air element.

+ Any pranayama works this element but consider retention on the inhale to feel the inwards and upwards movement.

+ Metaphorically, as air carries us, add Eagle, Crow, Aeroplane, or arm balances to capture the floating nature of this element.

+ Wind chimes are thought to produce positive and uplifting energy or qi. Their healing sounds can remove blocked emotions and stimulate creativity and inspiration. Consider doing a wind chime meditation. Concentrate on the sound of the chimes and their resonance. What do you hear behind the sounds? Music suggestion: *Australian Nature Sounds, Dreamchimes.*

To Your Life

Free-flow handwritten journaling stimulates stuck or blocked air. Clear your mind and clear the way with three unharnessed pages of writing about whatever crosses your mind. Like a written meditation, you acquaint yourself with your dark corners and your light, to bring them out into the open so they can be seen and heard. Through this process you clear your circulatory, whirring mind so you can put your attention to other things during your day[8].

---

[8] To find out more about this practice, go to Julia Cameron, *The Artist's Way.*

HOLDING SPACE

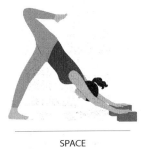

SPACE

The mind should be like an empty rice bowl.
If it is full, the universe can't fill it up.

ZEN PROVERB

To the Mind

Akasha: element of space or ether. Akasha is the most subtle of all the elements, the first element listed in Ayurveda

Chit akash: the space of the mind

Sense organ: the ears and sound

Chakra: vishuddha/fifth chakra

Direction: omnipresent

Complementary oils: oils from fruit and seeds, lemon, orange, sandalwood, tea tree

Essential vocabulary: unmanifest, subtle, container, primordial, emptiness, spirit, awareness, consciousness, receptivity, acceptance, perception, the source

Imbalance: shows up as spaciness, disassociation from reality, nervous system problems

QUALITIES OF SPACE

The qualities of ether, or space, are subtle, formed around an absence of all the elements.

- It is cold because it lacks heat from fire.
- It is light because it lacks the steadiness of earth and dry because it lacks water.
- It is stationary unless it is carried by the current of air.
- It is omnipresent, formless, expansive, and has no walls to hold it tight.
- It is in the empty, hollow, peaceful spaces.
- It is the barren winter.
- It is the void at the passing of life.

To the Heart

CREATING SPACE

We create space in our life by not rushing to fill our empty-ness.

We create space within the heart by willingly practising joy, gratitude, loving-kindness, and by inviting the heart to be more accepting of ourselves and those we meet.

We create space in our mind by sitting with ourselves, watching what arises in our thoughts in a non-judgemental, nonreactive way.

Space is the freedom between each breath.

When we create space, there is no limit to our expansiveness, to what we can take in and hold.

HOLDING SPACE

We hold space for another sentient being when we receive their feelings, thoughts, emotions, and actions in loving, non-judgemental awareness.

We hold space for another when we listen.

We hold space for another when we become present.

When we put down our agenda to fix what is broken and 'be' instead of 'do,' we hold space.

Space becomes the safe haven we create to navigate another's confusion.

And as we broaden and expand, we begin to see that what seemed like emptiness is pervaded with richness—a silent portal for everything to arise.

To the Body

❧ *Space* ☙

We are a product of space. In our human form we are 99 percent space. This space is held in our hollow organs, fascia, fluids, blood vessels, and cells. When we practice yoga, we work at creating and opening space within the body; by moving the bones apart, by softening the connective tissue a little, the body lets go of its holding patterns of tension and stiffness.

This practice works to create physical space with the use of blocks and invites you to insert sacred pauses and noble silences during the practice to challenge students to move from vigour to rest in a heartbeat.

OPENING BREATH

As you breathe imagine your body as an empty container.

Breathe into the nooks and crannies.

Breathe into the sides of the body, the front and back.

Fill your whole body with breath, right to the edges.

Nourish any emptiness with love and connection.

EXTENDED CHILD

1. Place two blocks at the top of the mat.
2. Place your hands on the blocks.
3. Press your seat back to your heels.

CAT-COW

1. Come onto your hands and knees with your hands still on the blocks.
2. Inhale, arch your back.
3. Exhale, round your back.
4. Repeat this for three more rounds.

MELTING HEART

1. Move the blocks forwards a bit.
2. Bring your hips over your knees.
3. Press into the blocks with your hands.
4. Sink your chest or chin to the floor.
5. Keep your arms active and lift your armpits away from the floor.

DOWN DOG

1. Tuck your toes and lift your hips up and back into Downward Facing Dog.
2. Stay for five breaths.

FORWARD FOLD

1. Look forwards and step to the front of your mat.
2. Turn the blocks up if needed, fold over your legs.
3. Keep your hands on the blocks and take five long, slow breaths here.
4. Press into your feet, rise up to Mountain, bring your hands to your heart.

Space

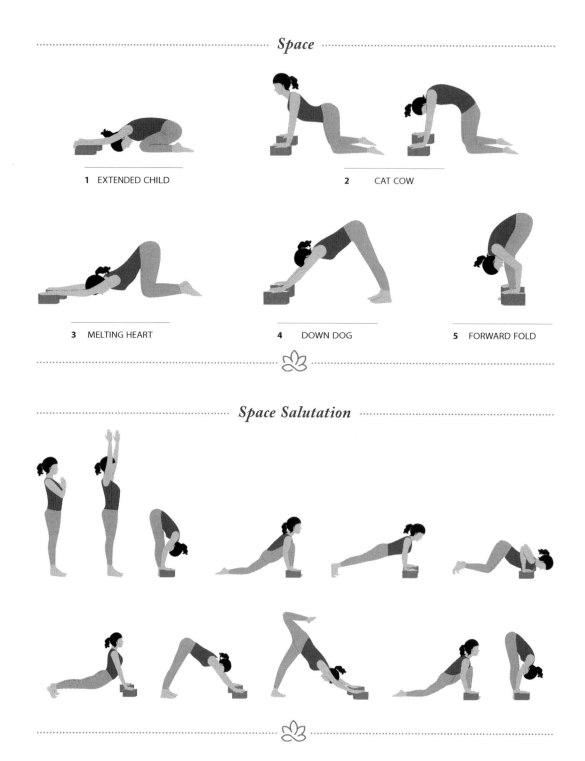

1 EXTENDED CHILD

2 CAT COW

3 MELTING HEART

4 DOWN DOG

5 FORWARD FOLD

Space Salutation

❧ *Space Salutation* ☙

Stay for up to five breaths in each of the poses.

Use the blocks under your hands.

1. Start in Mountain pose.
2. Inhale, reach skyward.
3. Exhale, bow, place your hands on the blocks.
4. Inhale, step your right leg back and put your knee down, look forwards.
5. Exhale, step your left leg back to meet your right.
6. Inhale, in Plank.
7. Drop your knees.
8. Exhale, bend your elbows, and lower your chest to the earth.
9. Inhale, press into the blocks, curve, and lift your chest forwards and up.
10. Exhale, press your hips up and back.
11. Inhale, lift your right leg into the sky, stack your right hip over your left hip, bend your right knee.
12. Exhale, square off your hip, step your right leg to the front of the mat, drop your left knee down.
13. Inhale, lift your chest, look forwards.
14. Exhale, step your left leg to meet your right, bow.
15. Inhale, half-way lift.
16. Exhale, fold.
17. Inhale, rise up to Mountain, reach for the sky.
18. Exhale, hands to heart.
19. Repeat on the left side.

Teaching Notes

+ As the practice begins, invite students to create space by
  - laying themselves out and taking up 'space' on their mat as if they want to fill the whole container of the room.
  - creating axial extension in the spine to bring more space between each vertebra.
  - lengthening the inhales or exhales or both, or extending the time between the inhale and exhale.
  - putting down any worries or concerns, to create space in their hearts and minds.

+ We heal from too much busyness in our system not by doing more, or trying to outrun the moments of emptiness, but by nourishing and honouring our pauses. The practice should reflect this by being slow and reflective. 'We need less, not more' is a relatable theme for most people.

✦ Grounding practices with plenty of props help calm and soothe the nervous system.

✦ Forward folds and inversions nourish the ether element and help create space in the mind.

✦ Blocks under the hands create more physical space for postures.

✦ Slow, calming breathing practices that produce a low frequency sound such as 'S' breath (as you exhale bring the tip of the tongue to the palate and make an 'S' or snake sound) and Straw breath (as you exhale purse your lips as if you are exhaling through a straw).

✦ Consider creating visual space by closing the eyes. This can be experimented with in salutations. Proprioception—or knowing where our limbs are in time and space without looking—works the ether element.

✦ Consider inserting sacred pauses of Savasana, Crocodile, or Mountain between the Sun Salutations, between a set of poses, or between all the poses, as an experiment. These poses will act as a punctuation for you to highlight themes related to letting go, creating space, or the duality of yin and yang.

✦ The unorthodox approach of inserting stillness into a vinyasa class may also highlight an unwillingness or inability to drop our busyness or vigilance in the middle of a class. Just as good vagal tone is reflected in the speed of the heartbeat on the inhale and the slowness of it on the exhale, being able to change from vigour to rest in a heartbeat is a good indicator of the tone of the practitioner's mind and heart.

✦ At the start of a class, Savasana enables you to set the mood for your entire sequence. At the end of class, it is essential for letting the practice download in the student's entire being, wiping the slate clean and settling energy before they arise back into their worlds.

✦ Einstein tells us that the thought we are separate from the universe is a type of delusion of consciousness. Question the notion that you are separate from the universe and there is 'me' space and 'you' space. Space is shared and omnipresent. It passes through us and around us. With your eyes closed can you feel a oneness or merging with all of life? Feel boundaries blur and a physical spreading and melding into the space you are seated in.

✦ The chakra for space is vishuddha, so poses that focus on closing and opening the throat, such as Camel, Bridge, and Supported Fish, work this element. (See vishuddha chakra.)

✦ Ether invites an expansiveness into consciousness. Connect to this through meditation or the primordial sound of om. Invite students to experience the space that lies in chit (consciousness), akasha (space), behind the eyes.

To Your Life

Sometimes when we have a problem, it seems so enormous and insurmountable that we feel there is no way through or around it. By giving ourselves space between the issue and the solution, often we get to see things for the size they actually are.

The 'Zoom Out' technique[9] allows us to place our stresses and unfinished business into the more expansive ocean of life. We are not trying to deny the intensity of our situation; instead, it is a moment to stand back and say, 'I see you in the broader context of my life.'

When we do this, what grips us softly loosens. By stepping back, we drop the story and intensity of the problem, and what could have become scar tissue becomes a little nick in our life.

ZOOM OUT

Sit quietly, maybe in a place that is away from your issue.

Feel the stress in your body. Where does it dwell? Does it feel like a niggle or irritation?

Note where it is located. Its size and colour. Name it for what it is: annoyance, confusion, sadness, indecisiveness.

Now step back as if you were zooming out on Google maps.

Look at the stress particle while floating above your body.

Look at the stress as your house on your street.

Follow this outwards path—from the street to the neighbourhood.

From the neighbourhood to the hills and sea that bathes and protects us.

Go on to the majestic mountains, continents, and the sphere of the whole world.

Find and follow your path through the stars and planets, ether, wind, and water, until you are a microcosm of the macrocosm.

Now look back; the original abrasion has become a little speck in the distance.

When we hold it up, it seems so insignificant compared to the incredible story of our life and who we are.

When you see it for what it is, slowly return—planets, stars, earth, neighbourhood, street, house, room.

Return to your body, at peace, lying on the floor.

---

[9] As taught by Dr. Scott Lyons.

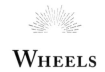

WHEELS

I see your true colours
and that's why I love you.

CYNDI LAUPER

Within every one of us is a rainbow of energy painted along the ley line of our spine, known as the chakra system. Like spinning doors, energy congregates and converges at your nerve plexus to converse about you and your life, where you came from, and where you are now. The chakra gateways line the spine from top to tail, assimilating, digesting, and transforming energy, working together and working on their own.

These energetic assembly points combine our life history and our present moments into a readable map that we can use to understand ourselves better and heal our wounds. It is from these centres that we can learn to balance what has toppled, pay attention to what we need to, and send encouragement to what needs to be revealed.

Each of these symbols is painted a hue of the rainbow and adorned with a lotus. The colours morph and change to reflect our true colours. Like the rainbow, there is no beginning and no end. Our hero's journey is to climb from the pot of gold at one end to heaven at the other so that we can begin again.

When all seven energy points are spinning in harmony, we feel at ease in our body, mind, and heart.

The cessation of their movement marks the end of our life.

❧ *Theme with the chakras* ☙

Compliment your chakra themes with the ideas and visualisations below.

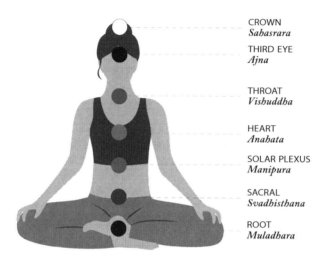

CROWN
Sahasrara

THIRD EYE
Ajna

THROAT
Vishuddha

HEART
Anahata

SOLAR PLEXUS
Manipura

SACRAL
Svadhisthana

ROOT
Muladhara

CHAKRA BREATHING

Inhale into the root chakra, exhale from the root chakra.

Inhale to the sacral chakra, exhale from the sacral to the root.

Follow this pattern, moving up the chakras until you reach the seventh chakra.

CHAKRA CHANTING

Move up the chakras and chant the seed or beej mantra at each station

+ **Muladhara**: lam
+ **Svadhisthana**: vam
+ **Manipura**: ram
+ **Anahata**: yam
+ **Vishuddha**: ham
+ **Ajna**: om
+ **Sahasrara**: silence/listen

COLOUR THE CHAKRAS

Move up or down the chakra focussing on the colour at each station.

+ **Muladhara**: red
+ **Svadhisthana**: orange
+ **Manipura**: yellow
+ **Anahata**: green
+ **Vishuddha**: blue
+ **Ajna**: violet
+ **Sahasrara**: white

AFFIRM THE CHAKRAS

Move up or down the chakras with an affirmation at each point.

+ **Muladhara:** I am
+ **Svadhisthana:** I feel
+ **Manipura:** I do
+ **Anahata:** I love
+ **Vishuddha:** I speak
+ **Ajna:** I see
+ **Sahasrara:** I know

ELEMENTAL CHAKRAS

Move up or down the spine and bring focus to the elements and what they represent.

+ **Muladhara:** earth, grounded
+ **Svadhisthana:** water, flow
+ **Manipura:** fire, energy
+ **Anahata:** air, love
+ **Vishuddha:** ether, purify
+ **Ajna:** light, vision
+ **Sahasrara:** no/all elements, union

TOUCH THE CHAKRAS

Move up or down the body placing your hands on each area.

+ **Muladhara:** sit on sit bones
+ **Svadhisthana:** one or two hands on the belly
+ **Manipura:** two hands on either side of the rib cage
+ **Anahata:** two palms on the heart centre
+ **Vishuddha:** hands interlaced around the back of the neck
+ **Ajna:** Anjali mudra to the third eye
+ **Sahasrara:** hands interlaced over the head or floating above the head

VAYU CHAKRAS

Bring attention to the pattern of energy at each chakra via the vayus.

+ **Prana vayu:** moves between anahata and ajna chakras as upwards and outwards energy
+ **Apana vayu:** influences the downwards and outwards energy from svadhisthana down to muladhara
+ **Samana vayu:** inwardly swirls between prana and apana at manipura chakra
+ **Udana vayu:** outwards moving energy around the throat and is housed in ajna
+ **Vyana vayu:** surrounding energy that flows freely through and around all the chakras

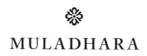

MULADHARA

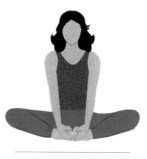

MULADHARA

A tree with strong roots laughs at the storms.
PROVERB

To the Mind

Mula: base, root, seed, essence

Adhara: grounding, stability, steady, safe

Called: muladhara, first chakra, root chakra, base chakra

Located: at the base of the spine near the perineum

Colour: slow, dense, blood-like colour that brings vitality
and nourishment to our bones

Yoni Mudra: Join the tips of your thumbs and index fingers to form a pear shape; spread
your other fingers and palms. Place the mudra with the index fingers pointing
downwards on your low belly. The downwards direction of the fingers draws
us closer into earth energy and the shape of the mudra represents the womb
or our first home.

Essential vocabulary

- bones, feet, toes, legs
- footprint, handprint, imprint
- earth, rock, foundations, grounded, anchor, drawing up from the earth, roots, taproot

- connection, tribe, ancestry, family, DNA
- instincts, primal needs, base needs, trust, fears, needs, protection
- support, survival, security, safety, flourish
- trust

GOVERNS

+ survival instincts, bodily instincts, autonomic functioning
+ legs, feet, muscles, hip joints, skin, hair, pelvic floor
+ skeletal structure, teeth
+ bladder, rectum, prostate
+ immune system, adrenals
+ intestines, digestion, elimination
+ nose and the sense of smell

IN BALANCE

- safe, secure
- grounded
- at home in your body
- feelings of having enough
- trust your needs will be met
- self-confidence, valuing yourself, present
- being okay with not knowing
- open to vulnerability
- trust life is safe

IMBALANCED

- fearful, insecure, 'flighty,' no sense of belonging
- a feeling of restlessness
- avoids things that need to be done
- lacks stability, can drift
- a feeling of lack or scarcity
- a sense of not being good enough/imposter syndrome
- displays addictive behaviour
- lacks trust

AFFIRMATIONS

All my needs are met.

I have a right to be here; I have a right to take up space.

I love and respect my body.

I am enough; I have enough.

I choose to let go of fear.

To the Heart

I long, as does every human being, to be at home wherever I find myself.

MAYA ANGELOU

Our journey begins here.

We start as a seed.

Like a historical taproot, this mula carries the energy of our pasts from one generation to the next, and within its kernel lie the joys, triumphs, fears, and karmas of our ancestors. It is our umbilical cord to our DNA, our primary tribe, our heritage, and it is the bridge between animal consciousness and human form.

Muladhara takes root at conception and develops in our first year. At birth, we slip from our primary home and into the arms of our caregivers as we prepare to create our roots here on earth.

The first chakra is the most important, for it forms the base from which all the other chakras will develop. Within this storehouse lies the genesis for all we will become and all we have ever been.

This centre is our psychological and emotional home and is concerned with meeting our basic needs or physical survival. As babies, our programmed survival revolves around receiving care. If the seed of this energy centre lands on fertile soil, we learn how to feel at home in our bodies and develop a sense of trust and safety towards the world around us.

If we spent this first year being starved of attention, love, and care, it is possible that in later years this void will become our verse of lack:

I am not enough,
I don't belong,
My needs aren't met,
I am not safe.

Tap into the power of the muladhara lifeline when you feel fearful, uprooted, pulled in many directions, or you are standing on the precipice of your life. The anchoring qualities he has will tether you back to safety and chaperone you away from fear. He will remind you of your centre, that you are enough and that you do belong. He is the life raft for your survival and a reminder of how far you have already come.

To the Body

❧ *Muladhara* ☙

This practice puts emphasis on building strong, stable legs to give a sense of stability and strength in our body home. The opening meditation is to help practitioners feel at ease and a sense of trust as they start to explore the first chakra.

ESSENTIAL POSES

+ Bound Angle pose, Child's Pose
+ Easy Seat, Hero, Thunderbolt
+ Tip Toe balances, Toe Squat, Toe Release, foot massage, pada bandha exploration
+ Chair, Tree, Mountain, standing Hand to Big Toe, Standing Head to Knee, Eagle
+ Hindi Squat, Low Lunge, Warriors, Goddess
+ Pigeon, Double Pigeon, Figure Four
+ Savasana, Full Prostration
+ Myofascial release and massage of the feet with a tennis ball or hands. Release of the calves with foam rolling.
+ Yin—Butterfly, Hindi Squat, Embryo, Dangling, Stirrup, Firelog, Dragonfly, Legs Up the Wall

OPENING GUIDED MEDITATION—SAFE

Lie down, close your eyes.

Trust.

Bring the soles of the feet together and let your knees fall out wide.

Place one hand on your belly and one on your heart.

Take a long slow breath into your hands and exhale completely.

Let the weight of your bones drop to the floor.

Continue to breathe into your hands.

Each breath sustains you and teaches you to thrive.

Each breath is a reminder that you have all you need right now.

Breathe into your body with love and respect.

This body, this life you have created, is your forever home.
It is your refuge, your personal oasis in times of need.

Go inside to a place that feels stable, solid, unmoving.
A place where you feel at ease and protected.
Sense its location, its colour and shape.
Take your breath to this place; this is your safe haven.

Life can splinter us, throw us off centre, at times call us in many directions, but this place within, your anchor, is patient and silent and always there.

Take a few more breaths into this refuge.
Know you can return here anytime you need.

Muladhara

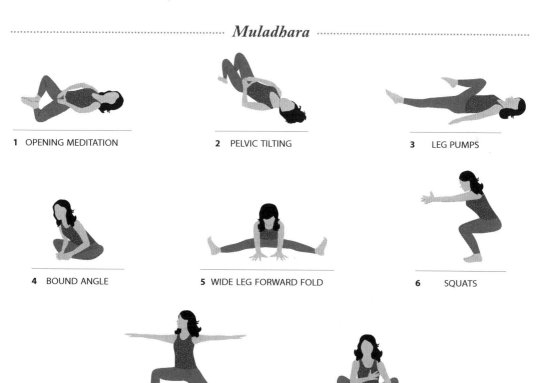

1 OPENING MEDITATION

2 PELVIC TILTING

3 LEG PUMPS

4 BOUND ANGLE

5 WIDE LEG FORWARD FOLD

6 SQUATS

7 WARRIOR TWO

8 HINDI SQUAT

PELVIC TILTS

From this position on your back

1. Bend your knees, and place your feet on the floor.
2. Place your hands in Yoni mudra over your low belly with your thumbs and forefingers touching.
3. Inhale, arch your low back away from the floor. The pelvic rim will tilt down.
4. Exhale, press your low back to the floor. The pelvic rim will tilt back up.

LEG PUMPS

1. Lie on your back with your arms by your side.
2. Bend your right knee into your chest.
3. Straighten your left leg so it hovers off the floor.
4. Switch.
5. Repeat this action, switching between your legs in a fast, pumping action.

BOUND ANGLE

1. Come to a seat.
2. Bend your knees and place the soles of your feet together.
3. Hold your feet.
4. Bow forwards over your legs.

WIDE LEG FORWARD FOLD

1. Sit your torso upright.
2. Open your legs wide.
3. Lean forwards and place either your hands on the ground or your forearms on a block.

SQUATS

1. Stand up.
2. Hold your arms out in front of you at shoulder height.
3. Inhale, bend your knees and squat down as far as it is comfortable.
4. Exhale, straighten your legs to stand.
5. Repeat for at least 20 sets.

WARRIOR TWO

1. Place a block at the front edge of your mat.
2. Place your right foot on the block and bend your right knee.
3. Turn your body to the long edge of the mat.
4. Repeat on the other side.

HINDI SQUAT

1. Take your legs slightly wider than hip distance apart.
2. Bend your knees and squat down towards the floor.
3. Place one hand on your heart and one on your belly.

Teaching Notes

+ Choose poses that connect you to the earth via your feet and legs.

+ Asana that heats the legs and brings blood to the thighs, such as Chair pose or Goddess pose variations, creates strength and inner power. When we practice this on our mat, it can translate out into our life if we feel adrift or ungrounded.

+ Consider the 'pumping' or hydraulic action of the feet. Lifting the medial arches of the feet or lifting the heels up and down in standing poses draws earth energy into the legs and pelvis.

+ Choose poses that create compression in the feet and legs, such as Thunderbolt or closed-knee Child's pose.

+ Concentrate on elongation and compression around the sacral/tailbone area.

+ Encourage the use of blocks; like foundations of a building they create stability.

+ Stay for a longer time in Tree pose, so students can explore coming back to centre when they lose balance. A block under the foot in the standing leg of Tree pose reminds students to connect into the earth.

+ A block under the front foot in the Warrior poses also reminds students to connect into the front foot, especially the heel.

+ Any poses that build strength in the bones, especially the thigh bone, fortifies the first chakra.

+ Poses in the lotus family, along with the Zen quote 'may we live like the lotus at home in the muddy water' connect the earth element to the water element of the following chakra, svadhisthana.

+ Slow, repetitive movements close to the ground will help bring the qualities of earth to this practice.

+ We must breathe to survive. Pay attention to cultivating breath presence.

+ The sense organ is the nose. Remind students of the tip of the nose eye gaze in some poses such as Upward Facing Dog. Before meditation, gazing at the end of the nose concentrates the mind and is said to activate muladhara.

+ Concentrate on giving students a feeling for being at ease in their body. Your language should reflect safety, okay-ness, acceptance of physical form, meeting their body where it is at today, and being centred/grounded. It should address gratitude—that we have enough, and there is no need to fear or feel we live in scarcity.

+ See Earth, Pada Bandha, and Hasta Bandha for more words and practices.

To Your Life

FOOD

Anything that grows roots deep into the earth—potatoes, kumara, yams, onions, dandelion root tea—is said to feed the first chakra.

Eating red food—such as berries, apples, tomatoes, and beetroot, which are rich in vitamin C—feeds the skin, bones, and adrenals. Adequate protein provides the building blocks of our body.

Eating hearty, healthy stews, curries, and chilli dishes warms the bones of first chakra deficiencies.

Sometimes an imbalance in the first chakra shows up in our relationship to food. Controlling what you eat when you can't control your world, refusing to be nourished when you need to be fed, eating less so you take up less space in the world, or overindulging in food can display as an imbalance in muladhara.

WORK-LIFE BALANCE

Do you bow to the god of busyness, plugging all your holes with work and striving to succeed? Take a step back and look at your intention behind overwork. Is there fear behind this—that you are not good enough, that you are an imposter?

PRESENCE

Do you tend to bury the holes in your life with wanting to take in more food, shopping, or stimulation? Being present and noticing where you zone out with overcompensating behaviours or addictions will help you understand your first chakra tendencies.

COMPUTERS

We live in a 'Vata Age,' ruled by electronics, and this can create a sense of being disconnected, as if we are living up 'in the clouds.' Constant scrolling is destabilising; we temporarily leave our bodies and even forget we have them under the screen trance. Earth practices help bring us back down and balance this airiness. Earthing yourself (walking barefoot), routines, bioenergetic grounding, forest bathing, hiking, and being in nature all help plug us back into the energy of the steady earth and take us further from anxiety.

CONNECTION

If you are feeling abandoned, lonely, or lost, seek out your sangha. A shared meal, a conversation, and group activities all help reinforce the connection to others that is our birthright.

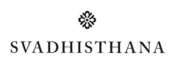

SVADHISTHANA

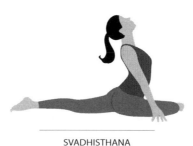

SVADHISTHANA

Energy cannot be destroyed, it can only be transformed.
ALBERT EINSTEIN

To the Mind

Sva: self, one's own

Adisthana: established and secure, her watery abode, a dwelling place

Called: svadhisthana, second chakra, sacral chakra, her favourite standing place

Located: three fingers width below the navel

Colour: the sweetest juiciest orange of happiness and hope

ESSENTIAL VOCABULARY

– sacrum—sacred, holy bone, hips, pelvic halves, womb
– water, fluidity, softness, go with the flow, current, waterfall
– creativity, expression, manifestation, rasa (flavours)
– pleasure, desire, longings, passions, sexuality, sensual
– emotions, expression of emotions
– replenishment, rejuvenation, regeneration

GOVERNS

✦ creativity, enjoyment, pleasure, sensations
✦ sensuality, sexuality, procreation, womb, menstrual cycle

✦ pelvis, pelvic chamber, reproductive functioning, genitals

✦ kidneys, urinary bladder, spleen, adrenals, testes, ovaries

✦ responsible for the movement of all vital fluids in the body, blood, lymph, salvia, urine, cerebrospinal

✦ social networks and forming relationships

✦ emotions and emotional balance

✦ tongue and taste

IN BALANCE

- creative, joyful
- energetic
- enthusiastic, playful
- forms genuine and balanced relationships
- sensual, can create real intimacy
- empathic
- generous, willing to share
- has emotional literacy

IMBALANCED

- shy, low self-esteem, body shame
- jealous, guarded, comparing, possessive
- mood swings, roller-coaster emotions, frustration
- rigidity of the body and mind
- averse to pleasure, lack of passion or desire
- acting out, attention-seeking
- lack of boundaries, exhibitionist

AFFIRMATIONS

I am a creative being

I allow myself to experience pleasure

I create healthy boundaries

I am able to go with the flow

To the Heart

Now that we have set the foundations in the first chakra—the conditions and boundaries for stability—we invite the flowing current of the second chakra to surge through us. The energy here invites us to step into flow, to move, accept change, create, and feel. Located near the sacrum, svadhisthana is related to our sexuality, sensuality, self-esteem, and ability to create meaningful relationships. The second chakra urges us to develop connections with the things and people in life that bring us pleasure, intimacy, and fulfil our yearnings.

Here we move from a relationship with the self to relationships with others as we reach out into the world and move from dependence to co-dependence.

As children, when our watery home is developing, we start to explore the world and our sense of autonomy. We experiment with pushing boundaries and building self-confidence. We begin to taste life through tactile experiences and learn what brings us pleasure and displeasure. These experimentations shape our personality and creativity.

Our desires—physical, mental, and emotional—stem from the power of svadhisthana.

It is the wheelhouse of procreation and creation, bringing into life all the working of our imagination. If we want creativity to flavour our life or we seek a life that is inspired, working with the second chakra will allow us to explore the art that lies within.

To the Body

❧ *Svadhisthana* ☙

Move with your breath and body in continuous flow while practising unleashing your emotional centre. This practice is a creative take on Single Leg Pigeon, sometimes called Swan in yin practices. The poses can be incorporated into any flow or as a stand-alone short sequence.

ESSENTIAL POSES
+ Focus on hip stretches and the pelvic region
+ Front of hips: lunges, Hero, Windshield Wipers
+ Back of hips: Forward Fold, Head to Knee, Pyramid, Triangle, Down Dog
+ Side of hips: Standing Half Moon Arch, Figure Four, Supine Twist, Pigeon

+ Interior of hips: Straddle, Bound Angle

+ Pelvis: Cat-Cow, poses initiated from the sacrum, poses that open and support the sacrum, extension and flexion of the low back, posterior and anterior tilts of the pelvis, poses that create space in the two pelvic halves

+ Myofascial release—glutes, quadratus lumborum, low back, sacroiliac joint

+ Yin—Swan, Caterpillar, Frog, Sphinx, Supported Bridge, Easy Seat, Child's pose

DANCING PIGEON

1. From Down Dog, lift your right leg into the air to Three-Legged Dog.

2. Flow from Three-Legged Dog to Upright Pigeon three times. If you hover the 'pigeon' knee off the ground in the flow, you build core strength.

3. On the fourth flow, pause in Upright Pigeon.

STRIKING PIGEON

1. Flow from Upright Pigeon to Sleeping Pigeon three times:

2. Inhale, lift your chest, exhale, bow your chest to the ground.

3. On the fourth round, lay your torso down into Sleeping Pigeon.

4. After a few breaths, move your torso towards the left upper corner of your mat for a lateral stretch down the right side of your ribs.

REVOLVED PIGEON

1. Move your torso back to the centre of your mat.

2. Thread your left arm under your chest and lie on your arm.

3. Turn your head to the right. Rest your head on a block if needed.

4. Open and close your right arm, joining your palms.

5. Optional bind: Wrap your right arm behind your back and grasp your right big toe.

SIDE BEND TO WILD THING

1. Sit up into Head to Knee pose from Pigeon on your right.

2. Exhale, arch the left side of your body down your left leg.

3. Inhale, sweep your right hand onto the floor by your right hip and lift your hips forwards and up.

4. Exhale, arch over your left leg.

5. Flow in and out of this three times.

DOUBLE PIGEON

1. Sit up.

2. Swing your left shin on top of your right shin for Double Pigeon.

3. Repeat entire sequence on the other side.

Svadhisthana

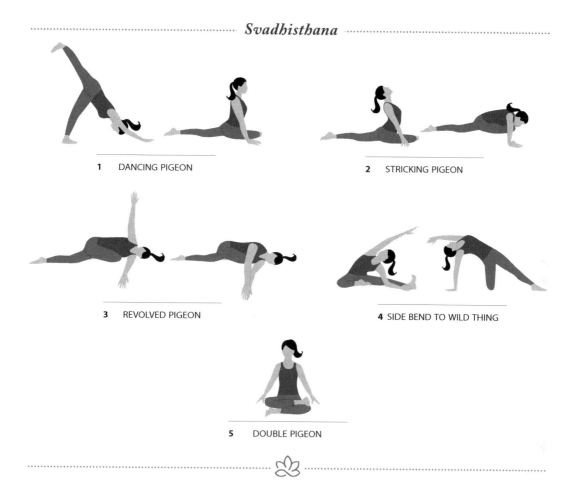

1   DANCING PIGEON

2   STRICKING PIGEON

3   REVOLVED PIGEON

4 SIDE BEND TO WILD THING

5   DOUBLE PIGEON

Teaching Notes

+ In chakra one, we connect the body to the breath; in chakra two, we ask how it feels to be in your body. Cue students to trace sensation in the poses.

+ Set an intention at the beginning of the class to visualise creating something of beauty.

+ Encourage students to follow their impulses physically when practising. Try introducing free movement during the class where students can express themselves without inhibition. Try turning on some music and inviting semi-guided flows. When we swim with svadhisthana, we step into the flow of grace.

+ Flows of all kinds suit this chakra—vinyasa flows, creative flows, free flows, circular movements, mandala flows, repetitive motions, tai chi, qi gong, and moving meditations.

+ Balanced svadhisthana people can change course quickly if needed. Many changes and shape-shifting during a class will highlight this skill.

+ Think of the poses as lubricating the hips. Use hip circles, opening and closing of hips, circular motions, Cat-Cow, and repetitive movements in and out of poses.

+ Introduce flowing fluid movements in Goddess, and the Warrior poses.

+ If a student's hips are open and they are falling into the poses, encourage hugging the outer hip points and legs into the midline to create more stability and containment.

+ Introduce the idea of finding 'pleasure' in the breath, the poses, in meditation.

+ Variations of Pigeon or Kapotasana
  - Supine Figure Four or Reclined Pigeon
  - Sleeping or Upright Pigeon
  - Pigeon with a block under the forehead
  - Pigeon with both legs bent at 90 degrees
  - Standing Pigeon
  - Mermaid
  - King Pigeon

+ Consider ending the class with soft rolling movements, such as Sufi Circles, after they come out of Savasana to leave students with a sense of 'go with the flow' in their bodies.

+ Lie on your belly and rock your pelvis side-to-side. Feel into the fluid, wave-like movements within.

+ Closing eyes during practice can help liberate those who have 'shy' movement patterns.

+ The sense organ is the tongue. Encourage a broad, soft palate during movements or in meditation. Try Sitali breath, which involves curling the tongue to bring this sense organ to life.

+ Tongue yoga. Poke your tongue on the inside right and left side of your mouth in a side-to-side motion. Invite students to contemplate the *rasa* or taste of their life. How do they want their life to taste?

+ Cue use of senses in Savasana. The taste of the inside of the mouth, the feeling of the clothes on their body, sight to the third eye, the sound of their breath, the sense of weight and lightness, hardness and softness, are primers for getting more in touch with how things feel.

+ See 'Water' for more ideas and practices.

To Your Life

FREE MOVEMENT

Examining your relationship to free movement will give you an idea if you have a 'blockage' in this area. If you like to be contained and colour within the lines, consider liberating your energetic creativity through Shiva Rea's Yoga Trance Dance, or explore the world of Gabrielle Roth's 5Rhythms.

Sensual movement, dancing, expression through your body, and fluid hip movements are medicine to free you of bodily shyness or awkwardness. Find a way to enjoy living in your expressive body. Explore bodywork, massage, yoga, and touch to bring attention to sensations and emotions that arise from touch. Allow yourself to co-create with your physical body.

PLEASURE

What is your relationship to pleasure?

Some people feel they don't deserve it and push bliss, gratification, or joy into the corners. By setting too many boundaries, or not letting people, food, or joyful experiences enter us, we turn away from feeling good about life.

Others overindulge in it. From sexual acting out, oral gratification, to addictions, the boundaries become blurred between enjoying the sweet things in life to actively living for the next dopamine hit.

What brings us pleasure is not always good for us, and what we deny may be just what we need. We were given our bodies to taste and feel and experience. Find the balance between indulgence and denial.

CREATION

What do you want to give birth to or bring into creation? What brings you joy? Mandala creation, arranging a yoga space or learning a new skill will bring the second chakra to life. There are many ways to create.

Allow yourself some unstructured downtime to tap into your expressive, inventive self.

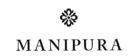

MANIPURA

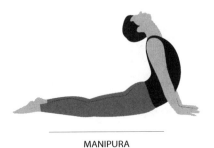

MANIPURA

Go within every day and find the inner strength;
so that the world will not blow your candle out.

KATHERINE DUNHAM

To the Mind

Mani: gems

Pura: city

Called: manipura, third chakra, solar plexus chakra, the city of illustrious gems

Located: his nucleus lies in the solar plexus, a pranic hub of alchemy and change

Colour: the yellow of the sun that burns bright to illuminate your path and give you the courage to follow your dreams

ESSENTIAL VOCABULARY

- metabolise, process, digest, assimilate, burn through, burn off
- alchemy, purification, transform
- power, strength, courage, will, determination
- fire, sun, day, heat, searing, potent energy
- molten, sparks, embers, bonfires

GOVERNS

+ adrenal glands
+ solar plexus, upper abdominal cavity, mid to lower back
+ digestion, metabolism, stomach
+ liver, spleen, gallbladder, pancreas
+ skin
+ diaphragm and the middle of the spine
+ eyes and sight

IN BALANCE

- has drive, determination, ambition, discipline
- has strong values and ideals
- feels life is in control
- sharp intellect, logical thinking and reasoning
- balanced self-esteem
- self-confident and has self-worth
- well-balanced digestion
- has purpose in life
- feels empowered
- good leadership skills, practical
- has willpower

IMBALANCED

- domineering, insensitive
- indecisive
- self-doubt
- lacks confidence
- issues with power, autonomy or self-confidence
- lack of self-will
- digestive issues
- self-centred
- overambitious, irritable, anxious
- strives for recognition, dogmatic
- anger that can rage or simmer if left unchecked

AFFIRMATIONS

I believe in myself

I am courageous

I have a sense of purpose

I release control

To the Heart

From form to fluid to fire, we arrive in the third chakra where we are called into action.

Manipura sits in our solar plexus like a glowing sun and connects us to our power, our identity and worth. In qi gong, this area is called the *hara*, the sea of energy, and our connection to the universal energy field.

As we leave for school, we snap ourselves off from the family unit and go out into the world to make a name for ourselves and shape the clay of our identity. We learn the story of what it is to be 'me,' and we start to set into stone our self-belief systems regarding what we are capable of. If we were programmed to believe we can or can't do something, we may carry that charge into our later years. If we were told to sit down and be quiet in our early years, the light of self-esteem might diminish.

However, we all arrived here with goodness to share, so our duty is to fire up this centre and discover that real power comes from stepping into the destiny that we were gifted and to shift our inertia into action.

Once we learn to distinguish what we want in life and go for that, the third chakra burns steadily.

When we stoke our inner fire, we learn to stand up for ourselves, but more importantly, we empower others to do the same.

To the Body

❧ *Manipura* ☙

This practice plays with Snake and Cobra variations and works at building strength in the core muscles of the back while at the same time compressing the belly.

ESSENTIAL POSES
+ Belly down poses, Bow, Cobra

+ Core poses, Plank, Side Plank, Boat, Upward Plank, Boat

+ All twists, supine, standing and seated—Child's Twist, Chair Twist, Half Seated Spinal Twist

+ Forward Folds both seated and standing, Plough

+ Triangle, Camel

+ Back and side body strengthening and elongating, Half Lift, Cobra, Plank, Half Moon

+ Myofascial release—roll a ball on either side of the spine in the mid-back and kidney area. Place a rolled towel under the belly and on top of the thighs in Child's pose.

+ Yin—Cat Pulling Tail, Child, Sphinx, Cradle, half Stirrup

Bhuja: circular coils

Bhujanga: snake

Anga: limb

Bhujangasana: Cobra pose

The snake makes its appearance in yoga mythology many times over: in the matted wild hair of Shiva, a belt for Ganesh, and support for Vishnu. In Kundalini tradition, it is the serpent that lies coiled at the base of our spine, waiting to rise and strike us from sleepiness to awakening.

The snake is known for its power to kill with a single bite, and for its transformative shedding of skin.

As the snake starts to grow, it finds its skin uncomfortable. What once served it is now too constrictive. The pain of staying in its skin is overwhelming, so the snake rubs its body on a rough surface to break the old so it can climb out and start anew.

And this is the process of transformation.
It becomes non-negotiable to stay the same.
We must move through discomfort, mess, and hardship
To be born again.

The energy of manipura is the same. It can strike with its sword-fighting tongue if cornered, or it can transform.

The snake postures keep our spine healthy and supple. When we lift our upper body from the earth to peer over our snake basket, we stimulate our solar plexus, massage our digestive organs, and awaken manipura.

SITALI BREATH

Sitali is a cooling breath. After a fiery manipura practice, cool the energy down with this soothing pranayama. The inhale brings in moist air.

1. Sit comfortably and enjoy a minute of Ujjayi breath.
2. Purse the lips and poke the tongue out, lifting the edges of your tongue like a curled leaf.
3. Inhale and draw a breath in like you were breathing through a straw.
4. Close your mouth and exhale through your nose.
5. Repeat this calming, cooling breath for a minute.

If you prefer, you can perform this by making your lips into an 'O' shape without the tongue curling.

MANIPURA MEDITATION

Find a way of sitting that makes you feel comfortable yet alert; a posture you can relax into while remaining attentive.

Take a long slow breath. When you get to the top of the inhale, sip a little more into your lungs.

Now let this go.

Again, take a long slow breath in; at the crest of the inhale, take a little more.

Hold the breath at the top without strain.

Exhale in one long steady stream.

This time when you breathe in, hold the breath at the top, try to relax the belly and the throat. Notice where the feeling of fullness sits in your body.

Exhale right to the end of your breath.

Let go of the technique and breathe normally.

Bring your attention to the jewel that lies above your navel and below your ribs. From here, your feelings of self-worth and personal power are generated.

As you breathe, notice if you are holding this area. Let your belly swell and fall, be soft.

Imagine the colour yellow. Let this fire fill your belly.

The burning light brings us the confidence to go out into the world and follow our path— our way.

Linger here, feel the experience and sensations well up inside of you, fill you.

(Silence.)

Place one hand on your heart and one on your belly.

Feel a luminosity under your hands.

May this day enable you to let go of the notions that hold you back.

May your every waking moment be a full expression of your divinity.

Say to yourself:

I am courageous.

I am whole.

I am willing to stand up for what I believe.

I am enough.

COBRA ROLL UPS

1. Lie on your belly. Tuck your toes.
2. Bring your forearms to the ground with your elbow under your shoulders.
3. Inhale, lengthen your spine.
4. Exhale, curl your chin to your chest as you peel your belly and pelvis off the floor.
5. Inhale, roll your belly and low ribs to the ground.
6. Repeat ten times.
7. Finish in Sphinx.

SINGLE LEG COBRA LIFTING TAIL

1. Lie on your belly.
2. Bring your palms to the floor on either side of your shoulders.
3. Press into your hands and lift your chest; at the same time lift your right leg off the ground.
4. Exhale, lower your chest and right leg.
5. Repeat on the other side.

BACK BODY COBRA

1. Lie on your belly.
2. Bring the tips of your fingers behind your ears.
3. Press into your belly and legs.
4. Inhale, lift your head, neck, and chest off the floor.
5. Exhale, lower your upper body to the floor.

COBRA BASKET

1. Lie on your belly.
2. Bring your palms to the floor on either side of your shoulders.
3. Inhale, lift your torso off the floor and look to your left hip.
4. Exhale, lower your torso to the floor.
5. Repeat to the other side.

COBRA LIFTING TAIL

1. Lie on your belly.
2. Bring your palms to the floor on either side of your torso.
3. Inhale, lengthen from your toes to your crown. Lift your torso a little.
4. Exhale, lift your legs off the floor.
5. Inhale, lower your legs to the floor.

RISING COBRA

1. From Cobra Lifting Tail, lower your legs.
2. Inhale, arch your spine in an upwards curving movement.
3. Exhale, lower your torso.
4. Rest.

COBRA FROG

1. From Rising Cobra, inhale, lift the torso, and hook your right knee up to 90 degrees to your torso.
2. Exhale, lower your torso and straighten your right leg back to meet the left leg.
3. Repeat on the other side.

Manipura

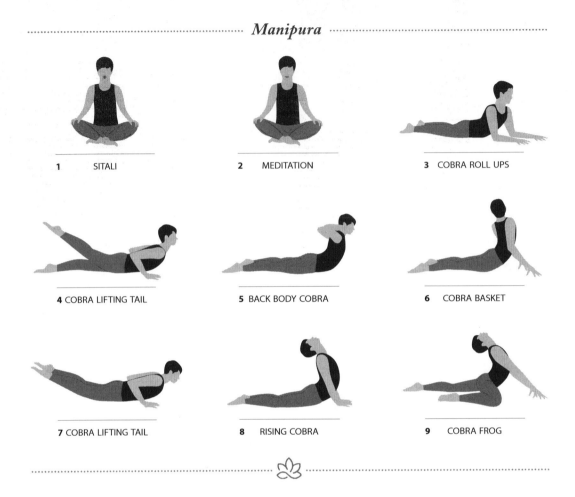

1 SITALI	2 MEDITATION	3 COBRA ROLL UPS
4 COBRA LIFTING TAIL	5 BACK BODY COBRA	6 COBRA BASKET
7 COBRA LIFTING TAIL	8 RISING COBRA	9 COBRA FROG

Teaching Notes

+ Focus on endurance or long-held poses to build heat.

+ Incorporate twists, compression, and elongation of the digestive organs.

+ Practices for the chakras can help stimulate the energy or tame it through either heating or cooling practices. Consider which approach you wish to take and why when working with this chakra.

+ After working with the deep core muscles, consider taking this power into arm balances.

+ Manipura is attached to mental acuity. The practices that stimulate the mind, such as Kapalabhati breath, will help clear out self-doubt and clear your slate.

+ Agni Sara breath or essence of fire will help digestion. This breath builds confidence and boosts energy. Try Sitali (below) for cooling the fire energy.

+ Teach the difference between force and assertion. Assertion is calm and comes from a balanced centre. Force is when we 'bully' our way into poses, our breath, and life.

+ Remind students at times to relax their belly rather than holding it rigid.

+ When you need to take charge of your life and regain your power, consider 'Ha' kriya. Ha mantra enlivens your self-confidence, strength, and worth.

+ Remind students that the sense organs for this chakra are the eyes, which includes how we see and how we visualise. Use drishti and meditation to explore the sense of sight. Encourage wide eyes like the Buddha—all-seeing or seeing the bigger picture.

+ This fiery hub's task is to assimilate, digest, process, and distribute energy, from the food we eat to our emotions and thoughts. A detox or rest-and-digest style class fits this theme.

+ See 'Fire' for more words and inspiration and Agni Sara description.

To Your Life

SELF-WORTH

Healthy self-esteem, self-confidence, and a belief that we are worthy reflect a balanced third chakra. However, our life is a jigsaw, and sometimes we lose the self-worth piece on our journey. What remains is a 'not enough' hole in the puzzle.

Not smart enough, thin enough, sensible enough, loving enough, strong enough, capable enough.

Our outer actions are a direct reflection of our inner belief system. The things we do, say, and consume mirror our self-worth.

We have the option to believe in our weaknesses and become embittered or work on our strengths and become extraordinary.

Every day we get to make choices, and these choices are in direct relationship to the value we place on our self-worth and our lives.

Reflect on your relationship to self-worth with the prompts below.

JOURNAL PROMPTS

+ What does it mean to stand in your power?

+ Do you feel people take advantage of you or disregard you in some ways?

+ Does it feel at times like your power has been taken away by others?

+ Do you seek approval or validation?

+ Do you have an ambition burning within but feel unable to take the next step?

+ Do you have a zest for life and feel like you have a purpose?

+ How do you return to the centre?

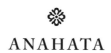

ANAHATA

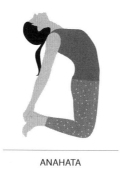

ANAHATA

To love oneself is the beginning of a life long journey.
OSCAR WILDE

To the Mind

Anahata: untarnished, unhurt, unbroken, the part of us that is unharmed.
She is the compassionate abode of mercy that lovingly tends to all matters
of love, kinship and connection.

Called: anahata, fourth chakra, heart chakra, unstruck—the sound that pervades
the universe, the soundless sound that arises from deep listening.

Located: in and around our physical heart. She is the heart beneath the heart.

Colour: the rich green of spring leaves.

ESSENTIAL VOCABULARY

– caring, nurturing, sharing, compassion
– altruism, generosity, devotion
– love, acceptance
– unhurt, unstruck, unbroken

GOVERNS

+ lungs, respiratory systems, breathing, ribcage
+ cardiac plexus, the functioning of the heart
+ blood pressure and volume
+ circulation
+ shoulders, arms, hands, upper back, breasts
+ thymus

BALANCED

- forgives easily
- feels kinship, harmony, and connection to others
- demonstrates unconditional love
- empathy, affection
- self-love, acceptance

IMBALANCED

- despair, insecurity
- loneliness, shyness
- antisocial, alienated from others
- needy, clingy
- self-serving, self-sabotaging or self-absorbed behaviours
- bitter
- passive-aggressive

AFFIRMATIONS

I love you
I forgive you
Thank you
I am sorry

Ho'oponopono, traditional Hawaiian practice of forgiveness and reconciliation

To the Heart

The fourth chakra sits over our physical heart and regulates its flow of energy. It lies like a bridge in the centre, connecting our outer relationships with our inner worlds. Anahata paves the way between our higher centres and lower chakras as she beckons us to cross from the physical to spiritual dimensions.

Anahata is said to develop between the ages of four to seven when we first venture out of the home to school and form new relationships. It becomes dominant in our life around the ages of twenty-two to twenty-eight, a time of forming loving partnerships, the meeting of life partners, and of heartache and heartbreak.

The love she contains is not limited to those closest but is altruistic love for all of our human family. In Greek there are four words for love: *storge*, which is maternal and familial love; *philia*, love for your brothers and sisters, friends, and those you know; *eros*, which is romantic love; and *agape*, which is a wide-open love for all beings. Like a compass, our heart can turn to any of these directions.

When this energy centre is balanced, we can forgive easily, feel kinship and connection to those around us, and demonstrate unconditional love and empathy. Our heart turns from being self-serving to all-serving, where we display an open-hearted graciousness to all who walk this life with us.

When this energy becomes imbalanced or diminished through sickness, loss, or grief we may experience a stagnancy in anahata. This deficiency may cause us to become shy, antisocial, and intolerant of others and ourselves. We may engage in self-sabotaging or self-absorbed behaviours. We may shut down outside connections to protect ourselves from further hurt.

If there is too much energy here, we tend towards neediness and may become clingy or demanding.

THE BLIND MAN

One day a woman was walking down the street, and a stranger bumped into her. She was furious. It was a hot day, she was busy, and now anger was pouring through her at how stupid and careless others were.

She turned to the man to unleash her anger, and when she met his eyes, she realised he was blind.

How could she be heartless to the blind, she thought in shame, and how could she overreact without understanding the full picture. She immediately apologised and vowed to step beyond her anger by turning it to compassion.

When we step out of our egos of anger, jealousy, and dislike, we can step into genuine feeling and acceptance for each other.

When we remove the blind spots to anahata, we can experience the faithful feeling that this chakra imbues—unconditional love and respect for all sentient beings.

To the Body

❧ *Anahata* ☙

This practice works towards Camel as a peak pose. Prepare the legs with standing poses and quad stretches. Work the upper mid-back with thoracic extension poses and side bends, and the arms and shoulders with binds.

ESSENTIAL POSES
+ Camel, Wheel, Fish, Bridge
+ Low Lunge, Hero
+ Gate
+ Cobra variations, Locust
+ Sphinx, Cat-Cow
+ Reverse Namaste, Cow Face Arms, Bound Humble Warrior
+ Myofascial release—Place a tennis ball on the front of the armpit/chest, under the collar bone. Place tennis balls on either side of the spine and between the upper, middle, and lower shoulder blades.
+ Yin—Broken Wings, Quarter Dog, Half Dog, Heart-Melting pose, Fish, Heart Bridge, shoulder flossing

BREATH OF JOY

Lift yourself out of lethargy or tamasic energy with this uplifting breath. Tamasic energy is slow, sleepy, dull and inert energy.

Come to standing with your feet hip-distance apart. This breath is in four parts.

Take a cleansing breath in and a long slow breath out through your nostrils.

1. Sniff one-third of an inhale to fill the bottom of your lungs.
2. Sniff two-thirds of your inhale to fill the middle of your lungs.
3. Sniff to the top of your inhale to fill the top of the lungs.
4. As you exhale open your mouth and let out a *HA* sound.

The breath has four arm movements that correspond with the four parts of the breath.

1. Raise arms out in front of you to shoulder height. (Inhale.)
2. Open your arms out to the sides so they are in line with your shoulders. (Inhale.)
3. Raise your arms above your head In Extended Mountain pose. (Inhale.)
4. Fold at the waist and bring your arms behind you like wings. (Exhale.)

Continue the four-part breathing with vigour for up to a minute.

STANDING BOUND FORWARD FOLD

1. On the last Breath of Joy, stay folded over your legs.
2. Bind your hands behind your back.

PUPPY DOG

1. Come into Tabletop posture on all fours.
2. Stretch your hands and arms forwards.
3. Keep your hips stacked over your knees.
4. Let your heart soften to the mat.

LOCUST

1. Lie on your belly.
2. Bring your hands back by your sides. Palms can be up or down.
3. Firm your legs and press down into your belly and pubic bone.
4. Stretch your legs back like a tail, firm your hands into the ground, and lift your legs off the floor.
5. Lift and fly your upper body off the floor.
6. Lift your hands and arms off the floor if it feels right.

BRIDGE

1. Lie on your back.
2. Bend your knees and place your feet on the floor.
3. Place a block on the narrow setting between your upper thighs.
4. Squeeze the block and peel your hips and spine off the floor.

ZOMBIE CAMEL

1. Come into a kneeling position.
2. Lift your arms out in front of you. Your hands will be in line with your shoulders.
3. Squeeze your legs together.
4. Lean back at a thirty-degree angle.
5. Hold in this position for a few breaths.

CAMEL TOES

1. Place two blocks on the floor where your toes are.
2. Place the tops of your feet and toes on the two blocks.
3. Inhale, lift and extend through your waist.
4. Exhale, lean back and touch the blocks on either side of your feet.

SEATED MEDITATION—HEART MEDITATION

1. Place your thumbs in your armpits.
2. Lift the armpits up, back, and down to broaden the skin on your chest.
3. Relax your hands on your knees.

HEART MEDITATION

The Ho'oponopono meditation is part of a larger Hawaiian ritual of forgiveness, gratitude, and love. By committing yourself to the words either internally or externally, you are taking a brave step towards your personal healing and therefore the healing of the world.

We are part of an intimate and delicate connection to everyone and everything. When we take responsibility, forgive, thank, and love others we remember we are not separate, and we make peace with the world.

Whatever you are holding on to, let it be released into the words of this prayer. As you repeat this over and over, feel the powerful energy within the words, release, purify, and uplift your being.

Sit comfortably.

Take your attention to your physical heart that lies left of centre.

Feel how it is cushioned by the lungs.

Now draw your attention to the bone of the heart, the sternum.

The next time you inhale, imagine you are directly breathing in through your sternum.

With each breath you fill the chambers of the heart like a life raft and your heart becomes fuller and lighter.

Keep breathing like this through the breastbone into your heart, inflating all four chambers.

As you breathe slowly, your heartbeat becomes less urgent.

Each new breath enhances your capacity to give and receive love.

Listen to my words and silently repeat them to yourself.

I am sorry.
Forgive me.
Thank you.
I love you.

Continue repeating these words I am sorry, forgive me, thank you, I love you, over and over again until you feel they become part of you.

Let their energy permeate your heart, your being.

When you have finished, sit silently in the vibration of what you have created.

Anahata

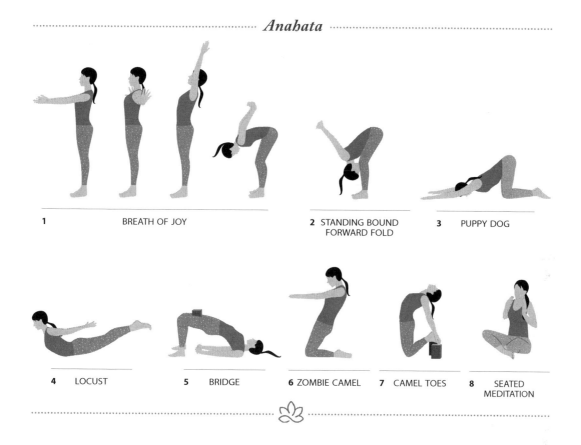

1   BREATH OF JOY   **2** STANDING BOUND FORWARD FOLD   **3**   PUPPY DOG

4   LOCUST   **5**   BRIDGE   **6** ZOMBIE CAMEL   **7**   CAMEL TOES   **8**   SEATED MEDITATION

Teaching Notes

+ Focus on expansion and extension (lifting) of the chest.

+ Experiment with non-traditional peak poses such as Bridge, Upward Facing Dog, Fish, or Camel and their variations. These poses will give you more time to explore postures in their entirety.

+ A class devoted entirely to Bridge and her variations works well with the idea of anahata being the bridge we must cross if we wish to explore spirituality.

+ When doing Cat-Cow, focus attention on the upper body moving as opposed to the pelvis moving.

+ The heart is the core of the body. The word *core* comes from the Latin 'cur' meaning courage. Warriors with a backbend element, such as High Lunge backbends, are both courageous and joyous.

+ Opening through the shoulder girdle and taking students through the range of motion of the shoulders will help open the chest in poses such as shoulder circles, and internal/ external rotation of the arms. Flowing, flossing-type movements of the shoulder blades explore any stuck points as they move over the rib halves.

+ Target chest and shoulder opening poses that open the pectorals and upper chest.

+ Target shoulder and arm strengthening poses.

+ Experiment with exposing breath on the back of the body in poses such as Seated Forward Fold. Note how the lungs cushion the heart.

+ Child's Twist and Tabletop help spread the shoulder blades and also complement back-bending movements.

+ The sense organ is the hands. Explore massage, touch, and partner work. The hands are the perfect vehicle for giving and receiving love.

+ Work on posture. Hunching forwards and collapsing in the chest are indicators that the heart chakra is blocked. Encourage pulling the shoulder heads back to open and spread the sternum and lift the chest.

+ Brahma Viharas literally means dwelling in the place of Brahma. These teachings are said to make up the core of Buddhist teachings which explore the four faces of the heart: loving-kindness, joy, compassion, and equanimity.

+ Metta meditation or loving-kindness meditation summons the power of love, support, and connection. Her words are, 'may you be happy, may you be healthy, may you live a life of ease, may you be loved.'

+ As anahata governs circulation, blood pressure, and flow, inversions will help her do her job.

+ Squeeze a tennis ball in your hand. Not only does this action feed up into energy lines of the heart but is said also to be about the same pressure that your heart pumps.

+ Pranayama reinforces the air element of anahata. Square, or sama vritti breathing, imitates breathing into the four chambers of the heart.

To Your Life

One way an imbalance can show up is wanting to please others or the desire for external validation at our own expense. Consider the word 'no' as being a sentence in itself, not needing explanation.

Be humble. Humility is a beautiful underrated quality.

Meditate on the colour green. Green is the symbol for new growth and potency.

VISHUDDHA

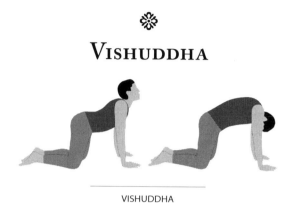

VISHUDDHA

The song I have come to sing
Remains unsung till this day
I have spent my life
Stringing and unstringing
My instrument

RAINER MARIA RILKE

To the Mind

Visha: poison or impurity

Shuddha: to clean, clear, or purify

Vishuddha will purify away any specks of dust that hinder our true expression.

He is the caretaker of our voice and the breather of life into our words.

Called: vishuddha, fifth chakra, throat chakra, purifier

Located: in the river of our throat and the soft pool at its base.

Colour: the lightest vibrant blues, the colour of the Pacific Ocean on a clear day or the sapphire sky in spring.

ESSENTIAL VOCABULARY

- express, speak, sing, project
- communicate, fluency

- truth, clarity, alignment
- swallow your ideas, lump in your throat

GOVERNS

+ throat, jaw, trachea, tongue
+ shoulders
+ thyroid and parathyroid gland, growth
+ breath and the voice

BALANCED

- inspires others through words
- speaks what is true with kindness
- able to listen to others
- easily able to express oneself
- open

IMBALANCED

- lie or deceives
- manipulates with words
- blunt
- difficulty expressing emotions and opinions
- reclusive or shy

AFFIRMATIONS

I use words to heal and empower

My voice is beautiful

I have a right to be heard

My words are important, and I am easily able to express what needs to be said

To the Heart

Stop the words now.
Open the window in the centre of your chest,
and let the spirits fly in and out.

RUMI

Now we move to the first of the higher, or spiritual, chakras. Vishuddha, which lies over the throat area, is the traverse we must cross to get from the heart to the head. The fifth chakra is our communication command centre. If this area is balanced, we are confident in our words and we feel safe in expressing our thoughts, visions, and ideas seamlessly without losing track, while equally being able to hear the truth of others.

The feeling of not being able to express yourself authentically, that you are living with words unspoken, of songs unsung, is something we have all experienced. Sometimes we feel that we can't communicate or find our voice. Sometimes we can't seem to control what we orally project into the world.

This chakra develops when we go out into the world, find our careers and seek success, which is reliant on good communication. If our ideas were silenced when we were young, or seen as unimportant, or we were taught to be seen and not heard, vishuddha may be imbalanced. The success and balance of all the chakras stem from good communication. We need to be able to ask for what we need, communicate with our partners, and express our will, needs, truths, and our heart's desires.

When we use practices to purify the container of our throat, we strengthen our ability to communicate with ourselves, and we form a deeper understanding of what it is that we need to put out into the world orally.

BLUE THROAT

When the deities and demons were fighting to gain the elixir of immortality, or *amrita*, they churned the sea so violently with their battles that the ocean spat out a deadly poison that killed anyone who came into contact with it.

Mighty Shiva was called upon by Brahma and Vishnu to come to the rescue by consuming the poison. When his wife Parvati saw him, she panicked and grasped Shiva's throat to control the spread of the toxin so he couldn't swallow the lethal fluid. The lethal fluid turned his neck blue and this is why he is known as the blue-throated deity.

Like Shiva, what we hold in our throat has the power to harm or heal, can be toxin or nectar, sword or salve.

To the Body

❧ *Vishuddha* ☙

The practice gives a new twist to Cat-Cow. Opening and closing the throat balances the energy in vishuddha. As there is a lot of knee work, take Child's pose or Down Dog between sets if desired.

ESSENTIAL POSES

+ Jalandhara bandha (neck to chest lock), neck stretches, neck cradling

+ Stretching the vocal cords with sound, japa mantra, kirtan

+ Cat-Cow, Fish, Shoulder Stand, Plough, Bridge, Upward Plank, Wild Thing

+ Eagle Arms, Cow Face Arms

+ Myofascial release—occiput release on a block, 'pinching' of the muscles on the side of neck, tongue stretches, roll balls down the side of the neck

+ Yin—Supported Fish, Sphinx, Snail, Dragonfly or Shoelace lateral lean with neck stretch, Legs Up the Wall, Caterpillar

STANDING DEEP BREATHING

1. Interlace all ten fingers and glue your knuckles to the underside of your chin with your thumbs touching your throat. Keep your hands in this position throughout the set.

2. Bring your elbows together as much as possible.

3. Inhale, open your elbows out to the side. Keep your chin level. Your palms will open and face the ground.

4. Exhale, lift your chin, bring your palms together followed by your forearms and elbows.

5. On empty, return to the start position.

SING—OM

1. Sit in Easy Seat.

2. 'Om' is sometimes spelled 'aum' and can be sung in three intentional parts.

3. Open your mouth wide. Sing the A sound from the back of the throat.

4. Round your mouth. Sing the U sound from the middle of the palate.

5. Join your lips. Sing the M sound from vibration at the front of your mouth.

LATERAL CAT-COW

1. Place your hands on the blocks.

2. Walk the blocks to your right side.

3. Begin Cat-Cow movements.

4. Walk the blocks to the front edge of your mat. Make Cat-Cow movements.

5. Walk the blocks to the left side. Make Cat-Cow movements.

CAT-COW BLOCKS

1. Put both blocks under your knees.

2. Place your hands on the floor.

3. Begin Cat-Cow movements.

CAT-COW ASYMMETRICAL

1. Put one block under your right hand and one block under your left knee.

2. Begin Cat-Cow Movements.

3. Repeat on the other side.

CAT-COW GATE

1. Come into Tabletop pose.

2. Place your straight right leg out to the right, in line with your right hip.

3. Begin Cat-Cow movements.

BIRD DOG

1. From Cat-Cow Gate on the right side, swing your right leg behind you, so it is in line with your right seat.

2. Take your left arm out from your shoulder, so it faces the front of the room.

3. Inhale, stretch your right leg back and your left arm forwards.

4. Exhale, round your back to bring your left elbow towards your right knee.

5. Repeat Cat-Cow Gate and Bird Dog on the other side.

Vishuddha

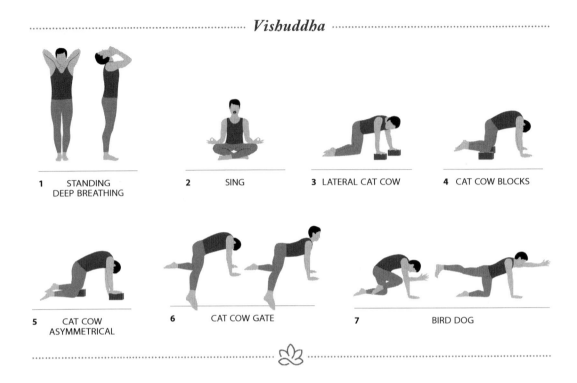

1 STANDING DEEP BREATHING

2 SING

3 LATERAL CAT COW

4 CAT COW BLOCKS

5 CAT COW ASYMMETRICAL

6 CAT COW GATE

7 BIRD DOG

Teaching Notes

+ Target flexion and extension, twisting, lateral movements, and axial extension or lengthening of the throat area and neck muscles.

+ When we lift the chest and hold it proud like a swan and fold our chin down and in, we create jalandhara bandha. The bandha is like a netted funnel that purifies the throat and anything that passes through it. It also provides a dam effect, teaching us to hold in what needs to be held.

+ Buddhi mudra is the mudra of clear, effective communication. Make it by joining the tip of the thumb (ego) to the end of the little finger (intelligence).

+ Ujjayi and Humming Bee's Breath both purify by creating a vibration in the throat.

+ The power of the voice can be explored through chanting and mantra. The Sanskrit word om is said to be a primordial sound or the most elemental sound of nature.

+ Cradling the head by placing it in the loop of a strap and around the foot in Supine One-Leg Hamstring Stretch helps release the guy ropes of the neck. This supportive head-holding reminds us to let go of the weight of the world.

+ Shoulder opening poses will open some of the muscles that feed up into the neck.

+ When teaching seated twists where you twist the neck to look back, include a twist of the neck to look forwards.

+ Singing bowls bring resonance and purity of vibration to the practice.

+ If you om at the beginning of class and the end of class, notice if there is more purity at the end. The practice of yoga is clearing you out.

+ Consider silent teaching with minimal use of cues and music. In a more established yin class, hold up the pictures of the poses.

To Your Life

STUDY—NONVIOLENT COMMUNICATION

Explore and study Nonviolent Communication (NVC). NVC helps us communicate in respectful, compassionate ways. Miscommunication, making demands on others, or not listening to what others are trying to communicate can harm relationships. Asking questions, avoiding assumptions, and listening well are skills we can develop to enhance all our interactions.

PRACTICE—THE SACRED PAUSE

During silence, we receive messages and recognise signposts. When we close down one sense, we attune another.

Some of us have difficulty in emptiness, feeling uncomfortable unless space is filled with actions or words. When we listen, we are only waiting to speak, and if we talk, it may be fast and overly wordy. If this is you, try to sit in the pauses and feel comfortable with the silences. It is in silence that we gain our most significant insights and in the quietness that we hear the truth.

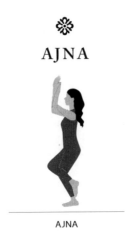

AJNA

AJNA

Your vision will become clear only when you look into your heart.
He who looks outside, dreams.
He who looks inside, awakens.

CARL JUNG

To the Mind

Ajna: to obey or follow, know or command.

Ajna is the guardian of the senses—sight, sound, taste, smell—and the witness of our lives. She operates beyond ordinary sight into foresight, visions, and the sixth sense.

Called: ajna, sixth chakra, brow chakra, the third eye centre, or the guru chakra.

Located: buried deep between the brows at the end of the nasal tract. She is the pinnacle of the lunar and solar nadis—ida and pingala.

Colour: the deepest indigo, a freshly picked violet.

ESSENTIAL VOCABULARY

- knowing, wisdom, intuition, higher thought
- silence, contemplation, meditation, turning inwards
- the third eye, witness, observer, seer
- introspection, self-reflection, self-study
- justice, ethics, conscience

GOVERNS

✦ between the brows, brain, forehead, nose, ears, face, and eyes

✦ pituitary gland, hypothalamus

✦ autonomic nervous system, growth hormones

BALANCED

- abstract thinking, imaginative
- can tell right from wrong
- discerning
- objective
- intuitive, telepathic
- insight, foresight
- perceptive
- clarity in thought
- realistic, self-aware
- psychic
- able to have lucid dreams
- wisdom
- spiritual awareness

IMBALANCED

- limited mental capacity, feeble-minded, or an unsettled mind
- dull, sluggish or confused thinking, feeling like you are 'out of it'
- difficulty making decisions and reliance on others' authority and advice
- indecisiveness or unwillingness to take responsibility
- disorders of the mind, fogginess, headaches, difficulty focussing
- not knowing what is real and unreal, hallucinations or visions or lapses into fantasy
- over-analytical

AFFIRMATIONS

I know the answers to my questions

I follow my inner wisdom

I act on my truth

I am a vessel for truth

To the Heart

The sixth chakra, ajna, is found at the third eye centre located in the midpoint of the brain, the domain of higher thought. It is here that we can tap into our intuitive, knowing side, and the voice of our higher self. What we perceive with our eyes, our thoughts, and visions are filtered through the projector of ajna. It is here the movies of our lives play out, so our job is to keep this lens clean.

Ajna is our guide.

The lower chakras all bow to the brow chakra, who is the overseer of their wants and needs, their worries, fears, and anxieties. Like a pilothouse, ajna looks over her younger brothers and sisters from the root to the throat, shining her beacon of light to usher them all to safety. She is the seat of the soul and the mother of all. This guru or remover of darkness connects us to universal intelligence so we can recognise the teacher within.

Ajna is the commander.

In Chinese medicine, this point is known as the *yin tang* point, the Hall of Impressions. Flanked by the pituitary gland in the front and the pineal gland towards the back of the head, these glands play essential roles in the modulation of night and day, sleep and wakefulness, just as ajna is the commander of vision and light. It is here we receive our dreams or visions.

Ajna awakens higher thought.

This chakra is most active between the age of thirty-six and forty-two. At this stage, we may move our thoughts towards more spiritual questioning, as if we were trying to piece together our place on earth. We may have insight or epiphanies about the meaning of life and existence.

Ajna is our guru.

When ajna is open, we see the future and become the navigator of our life as the noise of our confusion dies away. We understand what is right for us, that we have the answers we need, and we no longer need to look to the outside for what is right for us. Our inner wisdom silently wells up and takes charge.

It is here that we befriend the guru within.

To the Body

ꙮ *Ajna* ꙮ

The preserver of life, Vishnu, is often depicted riding on his mount, an eagle or *garuda*. A garuda is a mythical bird in the Hindu tradition. The 'king' of birds is known for its strength, vision, and wisdom. As the mount for the preserver of life, garuda can stay for the long haul in any situation. The Tibetan culture tells us he can fly without pause as he never tires.

Garudasana requires us to resolve to stay, focus, practice drishti, and concentrate.

This class plays with the metaphor of eagle.

ESSENTIAL POSES

+ Child's pose, Eagle

+ Standing Forward Fold, Down Dog, Dolphin, Standing Wide Leg Straddle, Pyramid pose

+ Seated Head to Knee

+ Poses with blocks under the head to support the brow centre

+ Myofascial Release—brow pull. Use your fingertips to pull gently between the brows in an outwards motion.

+ Yin—Dangling, Full Prostration, Crocodile, Sphinx, Child

May your life be like the eagles, riding high above the storms.

GARUDA AND AJNA

The eagle's sharp sight can recognise things from a distance, giving it foresight.

As hunters they calmly soar above life, always watchful and present; they oversee life with discernment.

As they have a bird's eye view of life, it is a reminder for us to stand back and look at ourselves objectively, becoming the observer, or the seer, of our lives.

Focussed eagle eyes are symbolic for being able to see the truth with clarity. Through the power of global vision, we can pierce fiction, seeing things for what they are rather than what we think they are.

MEDITATION

Sit comfortably, feel the four curves of your spine present. Let your sit bones sink into the ground and from this place grow up towards the light. Feel soft alertness in your presence, that sweet spot between ease and effort.

Interlace your fingers like a cap and place them on your forehead. This is the home of the sixth chakra. Feel the warmth under your palms and the lines of worry drop away. Soften the spot between your eyebrows.

Take a long slow breath into your hands and hold the breath for as long as it feels comfortable.

Release the breath and feel a wave of bright light shine and flood through the whole area in a 360-degree orbit.

Cup your hands softly over your eyes. Relax the muscles of the eyes under the steady warm heat of your hands.

Take a long slow breath into this space and hold it. Feel relaxed, at ease. When you are ready, let the breath go and drop your hands to your legs. Feel a spotlight of violet colour flood this whole area.

Ajna is the seat of your intuition, she holds the answers to your life.

If you have a question or a situation you are questioning in your life, offer it to the light of Ajna.

Sit in stillness and absorb any messages that come your way.

EAGLE CORE

1. Lie on your back.
2. Intertwine your right arm under your left arm and your right leg over your left leg, so you have Eagle Legs and Arms.
3. Lift your legs to Tabletop.
4. Inhale, stretch your arms to the back of the mat and your legs to the front of the mat.
5. Exhale, curl your elbows towards your knees as you lift your torso.

TWISTED ROOTS

From Eagle Core:

1. Keep your legs in Eagle.
2. Drop your knees to the left.
3. Repeat Eagle Core on the left (left arm under right arm and left leg over right leg) to Twisted Roots on the left (drop knees to the right.)

COW EAGLE

1. Sit on the floor or a block.
2. Cross your left knee over your right knee, so your knees are stacked.
3. Cross your left arm under your right arm, for Eagle Arms.
4. Bow forwards and rest your elbows on your thighs or a block.
5. Repeat on the other side (cross your right knee over your left knee and your right arm under your left arm.)

EAGLE TO EAGLE BOW

1. From standing, wrap your right leg over your left leg.
2. Wrap your right arm under your left arm.
3. Inhale into your Eagle.
4. Exhale, bow your elbows in the direction of your thighs.
5. Inhale to stand.

EAGLE WARRIOR

1. From Eagle Bow, unwrap your right leg.
2. Tilt your body forwards to make a T shape.
3. Keep your arms bound.

EAGLE WARRIOR ONE

1. Exhale, step back to Warrior One with the right leg.
2. Inhale, lift your Eagle Arms to the sky.

HUMBLE WARRIOR

1. From Eagle Warrior One, inhale.
2. Exhale, bow your torso inside your left leg. As you fold, undo your Eagle Arms and bind your hands behind your back.
3. Repeat the sequence from Eagle to Eagle Bow to Eagle Humble Warrior on the other side (left leg over right leg, left arm under right arm.)

Ajna

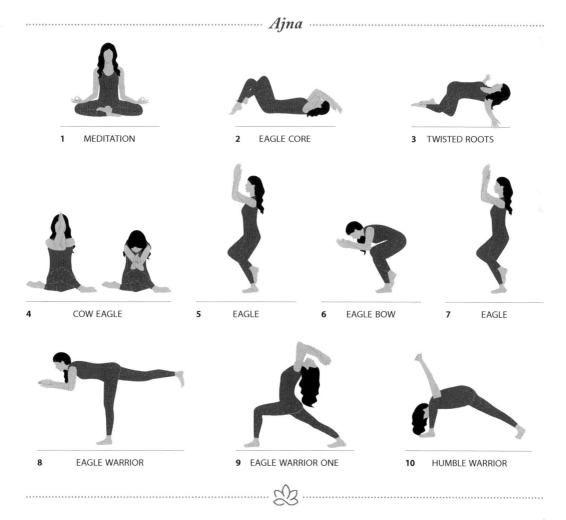

| 1 | MEDITATION | 2 | EAGLE CORE | 3 | TWISTED ROOTS |

| 4 | COW EAGLE | 5 | EAGLE | 6 | EAGLE BOW | 7 | EAGLE |

| 8 | EAGLE WARRIOR | 9 | EAGLE WARRIOR ONE | 10 | HUMBLE WARRIOR |

Teaching Notes

+ Ajna is the centre of attention; it captures all our thoughts, wishes, and desires. Therefore, we hold agency and feed it by placing our attention on what is important or of value. Pay special attention in the physical practice to where you place your body, your breath, and your sight (see also drishti). Set an intention at the beginning of your practice.

+ Garudasana balances the left and the right hemispheres of the brain, the ida and pingala, masculine and feminine sides. The third eye is the termination of the nadis. Choose poses that cross the midline of the body to bring balance. Nadi Shodhana also balances the energy in the left and right nadis and lights up the intersection of ida and pingala nadis.

+ Invite students into intuitive movement in poses such as Cat-Cow or variations of Sun Salutations; inviting students to move freely for a portion of the class is a reminder of their inner teacher.

+ Balance poses require an inner steadiness and concentration, which strengthen the qualities of ajna.

+ Poses that require you to look within—restorative, yin, and inversions—stimulate insight.

+ Closing eyes and taking attention to the midpoint of the brain stimulates ajna.

+ Emulate the qualities of the eagle: present, calm, objective vision, ready to spring into action, strength, and perseverance.

+ Train quietness and calmness of the mind with meditation.

+ Use Anjali mudra to press the thumbs into the third eye to stimulate and remind students of their command centre.

+ Kapalabhati brightens the mind. Like an internal brush, it will slough off debris, creating a clear palette to place new ideas and visions.

+ When the pulse of the mind is loud and painful, both physically as in migraine, or mentally in our thoughts, the medicine is quiet, dark, and still to help see and weather the storm. Similarly, keeping the physical practice dark, silent, and still will bring clarity to ajna to help soothe mental chaos.

+ Yoga nidra moves our brain waves into the receptive healing state of delta brainwaves. It is here we can receive messages and tap into our intuitive side.

To Your Life

THIRD EYE KISS

The philosopher Descartes called the pineal gland the gland of the soul. In some spiritual circles, it is believed that when you kiss someone between the eyebrows, you activate this gland, producing feelings of love, connection, safety, and security in the receiver. The hormones are thought to heighten our higher, intuitive self. When an opportunity presents itself, if someone needs guidance or love, gift a third eye kiss while sending a secret message of love and support.

YOGA NIDRA

Yoga nidra is translated as yogic sleep. In this state of enlightened sleep, we enter the transitional state between wakefulness and sleep where the body seems as if it is sleeping, but the mind is meditating.

During the practice, the brain waves follow that of sleep—moving away from beta, (active conscious mind) to alpha (a more relaxed, calm state) and theta, (associated with the dream state and R.E.M.), and eventually the delta state. It is in this delta state that the body starts to heal and repair itself, and we connect to a higher consciousness where our questions are answered, our intentions are realised, and our prayers heard.

Anytime we choose to heighten our awareness, we are waking ourselves up out of the sleepy states in which we live. Nidra sharpens the mind and stimulates the third eye chakra, allowing us to see more clearly and objectively and make better choices for our life.

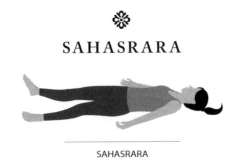

SAHASRARA

SAHASRARA

The grace of God is coming down upon us all the time,
like a gentle rain, but we forget to cup our hands.

KRISHNA DAS

To the Mind

Sahasrara: the thousand-petalled lotus, void, empty
Sahasrara is the confluence of masculine and feminine and the marriage point of Shiva to Shakti.

Called: sahasrara, seventh chakra, crown chakra, the thousand-petalled lotus

Located: at the fontanel, or just above the crown of the head, accessed through the sushumna nadi

Colour: the brightness of a million stars thrown together, floating above your head like the milky way

ESSENTIAL VOCABULARY

– spiritual, spirituality
– wisdom, enlightenment, understanding, realisation, liberation
– unification, oneness, being, transcendence, rise above oneself
– grace, blessings, divine
– light, luminosity, radiance, aura
– reach up through the crown, feel as if you were being suspended from above
– make yourself a conduit, let grace rain down on you

GOVERNS

+ upper part of the brain, cerebrum
+ pineal gland

BALANCED

- Feels a connection to all sentience
- Intuitive, empathic, connected to spirit
- Deep trust in oneself
- Able to access the answers one needs
- Can unlock the secrets of the mind

IMBALANCED

- Feels more knowing and above others
- May appear disconnected to life and others
- Lacks inspiration
- Closed minded

To the Heart

You are a spark of the divine

It is here we move from our physical realm to touch and unite with universal consciousness. Sahasrara floats above us like a halo, governing and overseeing our physical experience and calling us to connect into the river of love. He is the highway to bliss, or *samadhi*, and the gateway to infinite wisdom, inspiration, synchronicity, and connectedness. This centre becomes balanced only when all its sibling chakras are in harmony.

When we put down our thinking, analysing, and notions of separateness, we step into his web of infinite love. Through prayer, meditation, or silence, we open our attention to the god of our understanding, be that Buddha, Krishna, or Spirit, and ask that we merge with this supreme love.

Darshana is a Sanskrit word that means 'to see or glimpse.' We experience this when we receive a vision of the divine or we come into contact with a holy person or a deity. The mere sight of this person, or being in their presence, will bring us blessings and peace as they transmit their energy into our beings. We can also practice darshan by sitting at our altar with a representation of a beloved deity. By contemplating on their angelic essence, we invite in guidance and ask to be blessed by their revelations to help us on our path.

We see and in return we are seen.

ALTAR OF THE HEART

This is the altar of my heart.
A sacred venue.
In beauty and reverence, I place upon it
gratitude, in the sacred photos of loved ones.
A candle for compassion burns,
Saraswati dwells amidst smoke and flowers.
I let my intention settle here.
Anything I place upon my altar
I place upon my heart.

Place one hand on your heart; this is the sacred abode of all you hold true.
What do you place on the altar of your heart?
What do you want to preserve and protect and hold close?
Envision it, stow it there, make it sacred.
This love letter to yourself can never be taken away.

To the Body

❧ *Sahasrara* ☙

This simple acupressure practice prepares the mind for the state of meditation. The points are also chosen to help with relaxation, quieting the mind and therefore are beautiful medicine before sleep.

ESSENTIAL POSES

+ Inner work, silence, meditation, contemplation, concentration, solitude

+ Handstand, Headstand, Rabbit, Shoulder Stand

+ Tree with a mudra above the head or on top of the head

+ Head to Knee pose

+ Savasana, Yoga Nidra

+ Single Nostril Breathing

+ Chant om

+ Yin—the Rebound

BUBBLING SPRING—SOLES OF THE FEET

Bubbling Spring is grounding and useful for inducing sleep.

1. Sit on a block in Half Hero pose with your leg tucked behind you and the sole of your foot exposed.

2. Make a knuckle with your hand and massage into the point just inside your big toe joint.

3. Press with your thumb firmly into the point.

4. Yin: Reclined Half Saddle.

BIG WIND—BASE OF THE NECK

Big Wind is located just outside of the big tendons at the back of the head where the skull and the neck join. Acupressure here clears agitation.

1. Lie down.

2. Clasp your hands behind your neck with your fingers interlocked and your thumbs pointing down.

3. Lie onto your clasped hands and press your thumbs into the two spots. Use a firm, deep pressure or small circles up towards your skull.

4. Breathe deeply as you massage the area.

5. Yin: Reclined Tree pose, or Reclined Butterfly. Lift one leg into Tree pose. Support the Tree knee if needed. Keep your hands clasped behind your head with the thumbs pressing into Big Wind during the pose if you prefer.

YIN TANG—BETWEEN THE EYEBROWS

Massaging yin tang, situated between the eyebrows just above the nose, will clear 'overload' from your mind.

1. Sit comfortably in Thunderbolt pose.

2. Use your forefinger to massage the point between the eyes.

3. Yin: Embryo. Bring your knees together and place a block at the front edge of your mat. Place your forehead on the front edge on a block. If the block is soft, you can rest your forehead on the front edge of the block.

BAMBOO GATHERING—INNER EDGE OF THE EYEBROWS

Applying pressure to Bamboo Gathering will calm your nervous system.

1. Sit in Straddle pose.

2. Support your elbows on a block.

3. Press your left and right thumbs into the hollows at the inner edges of your eyebrows.

4. Yin: Dragonfly. Continue Bamboo Gathering for as long as it feels comfortable in Dragonfly.

100 MEETING POINT—CROWN OF THE HEAD

Applying pressure to 100 Meeting Point will bring calm, clarity, and creativity.

1. Find the centre of your head (fontanel).

2. Make a Mukula mudra beak by joining your thumb and fingertips together.

3. Tap the centre of your head.

4. Finish by interlacing your fingers and placing them over your head like a crown.

5. Feel the pressure on the top of your head.

6. Gently move the plates of your head around and notice the relaxation this promotes.

7. Breathe into your hands.

8. Yin: Waterfall, Legs Up the Wall.

MEDITATION—AKASHIC RECORDS[10]

The esoteric religion of Theosophy teaches that the Akashic records are a spiritual database outside of the human dimension, in Akasha. They store every bit of information about your journey, past, present, and future. They are said to contain the entire history of every soul since creation. The records offer guidance and wisdom to the seeker.

Sit quietly and at ease.

As you inhale, feel your body broaden from within; as you exhale, feel yourself surrender to all your life, your worries and concerns.

Bring your attention to the thousand-petal lotus floating above your head.

Feel the luminosity that arises.

As you inhale, expand the white light from the crown of your head to around your head.

Let the light start to fill up the area above you.

Feel the light enter you, your brain, your torso, your body.

You become one with the light. You are the light, and the light is in you.

Bring your attention to an everyday concern or question you have. Something that you are carrying with you on your journey. Something that you would like a resolution to or would like to know the answer to.

Seal the question in the vault of your heart.

In your mind's eye, see yourself stand up and start to walk down a forest path.

Eventually, you arrive at a large wooden door. Push the latch open and go inside.

Look around you. Many shelves are holding rolled scrolls. Some of the scrolls are tied with ribbon, some are old, some are weathered. Some are tightly rolled, some are loosely bound.

Turn around inside the room.

Scan the scrolls. One of them is for you, it has your name on it. It has the answer you need.

Choose your scroll, unravel it, and read the message.

When you have read the message, roll the paper up and place it back.

When you are ready, show gratitude for the message and leave the room.

Walk back to this room.

See your body lying on the floor.

Feel your breath in your body.

Feel your body in the room.

Start to make small movements.

Feel yourself grounded at ease and knowing that you have the answers you need right here in the vault of your heart.

[10]Inspired by the words of Cheryl Fenner Brown and Sharon Olsen. https://www.yogacheryl.com

Sahasrara

1   BUBBLING SPRING   HALF SADDLE

2   BIG WIND   SUPINE TREE

3   YIN TANG   EMBRYO

4   BAMBOO GATHERING   DRAGONFLY

5   100 MEETING POINT   LEGS UP THE WALL

Teaching Notes

✦ You can turn this into a full practice by starting with acupressure and following up with a yin pose.

✦ You can continue to hold the acupressure in the yin postures but feel free to release the pressure at any time.

✦ Create a vibrancy and warmth in your hands by rubbing the palms together before you begin.

✦ If you teach another style of yoga, consider doing an inversion practice with blocks and support under the head to bring attention to sahasrara.

Pressure can be applied through various methods:

- Pressing on the point with your thumb or fingers.
- Mukula mudra: Make the mudra by linking all the fingers to the thumb to make a 'beak' you can tap with.
- Rub: use your open palm or soft fist to make sweeping or circular movements over the spot.
- Open palm: slap the area with a soft open palm.

To Your Life

THE CHURCH OF SILENCE

Build an altar to yourself.

Gather flowers and incense, photos, mandala, and objects of love. Make it beautiful. Sit in front of your altar, your sacred space, as a practice or in times of need. In this place, cultivate respectful silence and listen with all of your heart. Be open to receiving from the network of the universe.

THE PRANA VAYUS

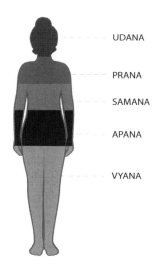

Pra: first

Na: smallest

Prana: the most important and fundamental energy responsible for the mental, physical, and emotional processes within the subtle body

Va: that which flows

Vayu: air breath or wind

The entire universe is constructed from Prana and within us this life force controls and regulates all the functions in our body.

Prana is broken down into five smaller units known as prana vayus; like faithful servants they move, direct and control the main Prana within our body. Think of them like currents within one body of water orchestrating and moving life below the surface.

Each of the vayus has a different home (chakra), personality, movement, and function.

In short they govern

+ Intake: prana vayu

+ Processing and absorption: samana vayu

✦ Distribution: vyana vayu

✦ Growth: udana vayu

✦ Elimination: apana vayu

The vayus make up part of our subtle energy body along with the chakras and nadis. This body can't been seen or touched, but our physical, mental, and emotional health and well-being is dependent on the balance between them all.

THE VAYUS, ELEMENTS, AND CHAKRAS

Apana Vayu: muladhara chakra, earth

Vyana Vayu: svadhisthana chakra, water

Samana Vayu: manipura chakra, fire

Prana Vayu: anahata chakra, air

Udana Vayu: vishuddha chakra, ajna chakra, ether

PRANA VAYU

Seated: in the heart

Governs: from the diaphragm to the throat, including the chest

Moves: inwards from throat to navel (inhale) and from navel to throat (exhale)

Chakra: anahata

Element: air

Imbalanced: feeling unmotivated, dull or lacking energy, restless or agitated

Prana vayu is inwards-moving energy. Easily understood as an inhale which enters the nostrils, presses the diaphragm down, and settles into the space of the lungs, this vayu is about what we take into our system. Drawing in air and taking in food, water, and what we absorb through our eyes, ears, and skin stimulate prana vayu.

It enters the head through the senses and works its way down into our heart and lungs. This vayu loves space to settle, so we need to make a home for it in our bodies.

When it is balanced, we have energy, we are alive, we vibrate and are receptive. We have impetus to move forwards and gather ideas.

Loud, constant, and overwhelming sensory stimulation can cause an overload. When this wee wind is out of balance, like an eddy, our minds become restless, anxious, and agitated, our attention impulsive. If the energy doesn't have a home, it gathers itself like tumbleweed and scatters everywhere not knowing where to land.

We can feed this vayu with meditation to create space and quietness. When we feed ourselves with beautiful sensory input, use our senses to invite in healing colours, tastes, sounds, and vision, we calm and balance the inner wind of vayu.

IN PRACTICE

+ Asana: backbends and inversions to open heart and lungs

+ Breath: antar kumbhaka—retention of the breath at the top of the inhale

+ Mudra: Prana mudra, join the tips of the ring finger and the little finger to the thumb. Stretch out the index and middle fingers.

+ Meditation and Savasana: create space for prana to flow in our minds

APANA VAYU

Seated: in the low belly

Governs: low belly down, including pelvis, pelvic floor, digestive organs, legs and feet. It overseas elimination and bringing new life into the world through childbirth

Moves: down and out mainly from the navel to the pelvis

Chakra: muladhara

Element: earth

Imbalanced: feeling ungrounded, blocked or stuck, digestive issues, lack of confidence, menstrual problems

Apana vayu functions mainly in the low belly and pelvic floor and within the reproductive and digestive organs. Its downward and outward movement is responsible for elimination of everything we take in and it's balance is indicated by our willingness to let go. This earth bound energy cleanses our body, eliminates what we don't need, and helps to give birth to new life. It is a grounding and stabilising energy.

IN PRACTICE

+ Asana: Squat, poses that work the legs and feet such as Warrior poses, Virasana

+ Breath: bahya kumbhaka—retention of the breath at the end of the exhale. Long, slow exhales with an audible sigh. Lengthening the exhales.

+ Mudra: apana mudra for releasing negative thoughts, emotions, and energy that is not serving you. Apana mudra is performed by bending the middle finger, the ring finger, and the thumb so that the tips of these fingers are touching. The index finger and little finger remain straight. This mudra is usually practiced with both hands.

+ Mula Bandha: subtle and soft practice with mula bandha will engage apana. Hold and stabilise it at the root by gently squeezing perineum, thereby redirecting the energy we need back into our body.

+ Sandbags to ground you to earth's energy

Prana and apana work hand in hand. In tandem they regulate the incoming and outgoing energy, the root and apex of our body.

When we inhale prana vayu moves from the core up and apana moves from the core down. When we exhale they move in opposite directions, meeting in the middle.

UDANA VAYU

Seated: throat

Governs: throat and head, all sensory function and growth, speech

Moves: upwards and outwards expellation of air from the throat to the head

Chakra: vishuddha and moves up to ajna

Element: ether or space

Imbalanced: difficulty with speech, unable to articulate, problems with throat and neck, difficulty breathing, respiratory conditions, stress and tension

Udana vayu is the upwards and outwards wind of communication active around the heart to the head. It rules the throat and if in balance we can say what we mean or put what we think out into the world with kind expression. It works in conjunction with the other vayus, so if they are in balance, udana will also be at ease. Responsible for upwards lift and upwards movement, this vayu is connected with physical growth, reaching for lofty goals—it helps us hold our heads up high and to stand tall and strong.

IN PRACTICE

✦ Asana: Crow pose for its uplifting quality, inversions that direct energy to the head and neck such as Shoulder Stand. Poses that create space and lift in the spine.

✦ Breath: Brahmari or Bee's breath (inhale, then humm a long exhale).

✦ Mudra: Udana mudra, join the tip of the index, middle and ring finger to the thumb. Extend the little finger.

✦ Bhanda: jalandhara

✦ Chanting: Om brings emphasis to the throat, mantra and chanting

✲

SAMANA VAYU

Seated: navel

Governs: the area between the navel and solar plexus, metabolism, digestive fire

Moves: inwards from the periphery to the core

Chakra: manipura

Element: fire

Imbalanced: digestive issues, worrying, inability to discern, holding on to toxins in body, unable to make sound judgements

Samana vayu flows in an inwards, circular motion from the periphery to the core. It governs the navel centre and organs of digestion, it equalises and balances all we take in and ingest—taking information, food, and energy from the outside right into the centre of our being. Here it is processed, sorted, metabolised, and distributed to feed all aspects of our life.

Imbalances in the vayu show up as a weak or overactive digestion, loss of appetite, or the inability to process difficult situations in our life. This vayu can be aggravated by worry, fear, and stress, which sit in our belly churning the energy in our 'second' brain.

This centre can be balanced by drawing upwards and downwards energy to meet in our centre.

In balance we feel centred and strong and discerning.

IN PRACTICE

+ Asana: any postures that pull energy to the core, twists and forward folds

+ Breath: Sama Vritti—the middle path of breathing, inhales and exhales are even in length, balances the energy of prana and apana. Forceful exhales to move air out such as Kapalabhati.

+ Mudra: Samana mudra is also called Mukula mudra. Join all the fingers to the tip of the thumbs on both hands.

+ Uddiyana bhanda: Upward Flying Lock, pulls digestive organs in and up

Uddiyana Bhanda: Upward Flying Lock

Ud: upwards

Uddiyana bhanda works to pull the navel contents, the organs of digestion, in and up while keeping a strong and straight spine. This allows an unobstructed flow of energy from the pelvis up the spine. The Hatha Yoga Pradipika says this breath encourages flow in the sushumna nadi or central channel and by practising it you will conquer death and become young again.

1. Stand with your feet a little wider than hip distance apart.
2. Inhale, lift your arms up.
3. Exhale, bend your knees, place hands on thighs, and bring your weight forwards a bit into your hands.
4. At the end of the exhale, hold the breath out and pull the belly in and up as if you were trying to vacuum it under the low ribs.
5. Keep your jaw soft and lungs relaxed.
6. Hold your belly in on the no breath for a count of four or five.
7. Release the belly and the diaphragm then inhale.
8. Stand up.
9. Try to keep the throat soft and avoid hardening or gripping.

VYANA VAYU

Seated: pervades our entire body from the navel out, runs through all the nadis

Governs: circulation and connection of all body processes, coordination and movement manifests on the skin or the periphery, pumping of the heart

Moves: from the centre outwards

Chakra: no particular chakra but more associated with svadhisthana

Element: water

Imbalanced: feeling of incoordination or lack of cohesion or wholeness, feeling disjointed in the body and mind

Vyana vayu moves in all directions throughout our body circulating blood, lymph, nutrients, and prana. Through the beat of the heart this vayu moves and pulses from the core of the body to the periphery like a river in an outwards spiral motion. Governing the circulatory and peripheral nervous system, it circulates and distributes prana through our energetic pathways, removing blockages or stagnation that may result in ill health.

Imbalances in this vayu may show up as circulation disorders, heart issues, and blocked arteries. Thoughts and feelings circulate on this vayu, so in balance our thoughts and emotions flow freely. But as this vayu is pervasive and touches everything within us the problems can travel throughout the whole body.

IN PRACTICE

+ Asana: standing poses, vinyasa to encourage circulation and movement of lymph, Sun Salutations, Savasana

+ Breath: Nadi Shodhana: with focus on expanding the lungs and chest as you breath in

+ Mudra: Vyana mudra. Join the tip of the index and middle finger to the thumb. Extend the ring and little fingers.

FLOW WITH THE DEITIES

Yesterday is gone, tomorrow has not yet come, we only have today. Let us begin.

MOTHER THERESA

Now that we are warmed up, we can balance, flow, or stand firm into the warrior's heart.

This section brings to life the gods and goddesses of Hindu mythology. When we respect, honour, and pay homage to what they represent, we invoke that spirit into our lives. Each of the deities and their avatars represents various qualities and aspects that lie within us and our lives.

THE TRIMURTI

The trimurti, or trinity, are the three principal figures that are worshipped in Hinduism.

Brahma is the creator. He is the supreme being who has done his work through the gift of creation. His feminine counterpart is Saraswati, the goddess of learning.

Vishnu is the preserver. As the middleman, Vishnu's role is to maintain order amidst the chaos of creations from Brahma and the destruction of it all from Shiva. His avatars or human incarnations are Krishna and Rama. His feminine counterpart is Lakshmi, the goddess of wealth and beauty.

Shiva is the destroyer. His destruction is necessary to start the cycle again. He represents the end of the journey and new beginnings. His feminine counterpart is Shakti, who takes many forms: Parvarti, Kali, and Durga.

Generate

Organise

Destroy

Theme with the deities

Devi or **deva**: shining one

As well as the trimurti, Hinduism and Buddhism are adorned with mythical gods and goddesses that represent aspects of ourselves that we would like to access or bring into the light. A deity is an energetic representation of the qualities we seek— love, compassion, gratitude or acceptance.

Immersing ourselves in Kali, Tara, Ganesha, or the deity of choice is to call up their powers and invoke their qualities when we need help or guidance or when we wish to embody their attributes.

Theming with the deities is a relatable way to apply yoga philosophy into your class and can be done through story, poses, qualities, mantra, or mudras. Below are some of the more famous characters and their qualities.

- ✦ Courage or confidence: Kali, Durga, Hanuman
- ✦ Compassion: Kali
- ✦ Compassion and healing: Tara
- ✦ Grounding: Ganesha
- ✦ Embracing change: Shiva
- ✦ Balance of strength and softness: Parvarti
- ✦ To move through roadblocks: Ganesha, Shiva
- ✦ Protection: Durga
- ✦ Abundance, manifestion, fortunes, and romance: Lakshmi
- ✦ Communication, learning, wisdom, and study: Saraswati

HANUMAN THE HERO

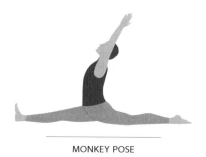

MONKEY POSE

Whenever you find yourself doubting how far you can go,
just remember how far you have come. Remember everything you have faced,
all the battles you have won, and all the fears you have overcome.

UNKNOWN

To the Mind

Hanuman: means 'broken jaw.'

He is the monkey-faced god, revered for his dexterity and strength, born to mother Anjana and father Kesari, he is also associated with Vayu, the god of wind. A *bhakti* (devotional) yogi, dedicated to the love of his guru Ram, Hanuman represents pure love and devotion.

The pose Hanumanasana is the combination of the Forward Splits and Anjaneyasana, the Lunge.

To the Heart

THE RESCUE OF SITA

Hanuman the playful, curious monkey seemed to be endlessly getting into mischief. He loved nothing more than to swing in the trees devouring fruit. One day in excitement, Hanuman mistook the sun for a big juicy mango. He jumped to the sun but was struck back to Earth by Indra, the lord of the sky and lightning. As he fell to the ground, his jaw smashed, which gave rise to his name, Hanuman, meaning broken jaw.

For the first time, this intelligent, mighty monkey forgot who he was. Hanuman felt weak and powerless; he had lost his purpose and strength. Hanuman was taken deep into the forest to recover, to live with an army of brilliant shapeshifter monkeys. Here he learnt the power of devotional love when he met his guru Ram and his beloved Sita. He would do anything, without exception, to serve them.

One day Sita was abducted. The monkey clan hatched a plan for her rescue. All the monkeys gathered to urge Hanuman to make the giant leap to Lanka to claim back Sita. Cursed as a little monkey boy for his mischievous meddling ways, Hanuman had forgotten his divinity and was clouded by doubt.

The other monkeys urged him on: 'Hanuman, Hanuman, you are the son of the god of wind, you have the power and strength within you to make the great leap.'

Upon remembering his power, his higher self, and his great love for Ram, he leapt across the great divide to rescue Sita and reunite her with Ram.

MANTRA
Namo…Namo…Anjaninandanaaya
Jaya Seeyaa Raama, Jai Jai Hanuman
I bow, I bow again and again to Anjani's son, Hanuman
Victory to Sita and Ram, victory to Hanuman
Victory over the darkness of suffering[11]

---

[11] Mantra and translation courtesy of Krisha Das. Reprinted with permission.
https://www.krishnadas.com/lyrics/baba-hanuman/

To the Body

⤷ *Flying Monkey* ⤶

Focusing on the hamstrings and hip flexors, these flows warm the component body parts towards the peak pose of Hanumanasana, or Monkey pose.

BEGINNING BREATH—HERO BREATH

Hanuman's spiritual father Vayu, enraged at seeing his son cast to the ground by Indra, drew in a big breath and captured all of life on his inhale. All the gods panicked, saying to Vayu: 'Release, release; we can't breathe anymore. Please put life back into our earth.' At some point, he exhaled, and the wind of his breath flooded the earth.

This practice imitates the breath of Vayu, when he inhaled the world into him.

During the suspension, or kumbhaka, sit with ease, relax into not knowing without force.

Relax the shoulders and base of the throat.

This is the state of *antara kumbhaka*, which means 'full container.'

Some of us need to inhale into our life, to take in more sustenance and support; some of us need to exhale, to let go a little. Which breath do you need to pay attention to today?

1. Sit comfortably.
2. Inhale to your full capacity through both nostrils.
3. Open the mouth and let out a long *haaaaaaa* sound, like a sigh.
4. Inhale to full; hold the breath for a count of four or five.
5. Exhale through both nostrils.
6. Repeat. This time, suspend the breath a little longer at the top.
7. Let go of the breath if you feel a strain arising around the throat.
8. Continue to breathe in this way for a minute.
9. Sit in the resonance of what you have created.

+ Flow One: Low Lunge to Half Splits (three times)

+ Flow Two: Runner's Lunge to Pyramid pose (three times), Low Lunge Bind

+ Flow Three: Crescent Lunge to Aeroplane to Half Moon to Warrior Two to Triangle

+ Flow Four: Crescent Lunge to Crescent Lunge with Eagle Arms to Warrior Three with Eagle Arms to Standing Splits to Crescent Lunge

Flying Monkey

FLOW ONE

1(X3) LOW LUNGE HALF SPLITS   **2** VINYASA

FLOW TWO

1(X3) RUNNER'S PYRAMID   **2** LOW LUNGE
LUNGE   POSE   BIND

FLOW THREE

1 CRESCENT LUNGE   **2** AEROPLANE   **3** HALF MOON   **4** WARRIOR TWO   **5** TRIANGLE

FLOW FOUR

1 CRESCENT LUNGE   **2** EAGLE ARMS   **3** WARRIOR THREE   **4** STANDING SPLITS   **5** CRESCENT LUNGE
EAGLE ARMS

Teaching Notes

✦ You can expand the flows above by adding a vinyasa after each set, (High Plank, Low Plank, Up Dog, Down Dog.)

✦ The theme of Hanuman works with any themes associated with love or devotion.

✦ Pair up the qualities of Hanuman with Virasana or Hero's pose. Vira means 'hero' or 'brave.' Hanuman is both hero and servant to his beloved Lord Rama. In Hero pose, Hanuman is pictured sitting at the king's feet in a gesture of adoration, humbleness, and servitude. He is also depicted seated in Half Hero pose and Half Squat. His hands are clawing open the skin over his heart to reveal Rama and Sita.

To Your Life

BRING ON THE BHAKTI

Hanuman was devoted to his beloved Ram. He understood that to love others fully is more powerful and enriching than to be the beloved. Hanuman was a bhakti yogi—he loved for love's sake and stood in service to Ram. He worshipped and adored him.

We all worship or are devoted to something or someone. Who or what we choose to adore will be where we put our energy and attention.

To serve without wanting anything in return is a practice we can take on in our daily life. From the simple acts of cooking and cleaning for others to community service, consider finding a way that you can serve for the sake of it.

When we use our life force to love and fulfil our duties, we reach our highest potential as humans.

We become heroes of our own life.

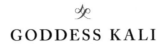

GODDESS KALI

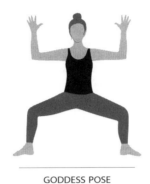

GODDESS POSE

Kali understands that the greatest of all love arises from our capacity to help others walk through their fires while at the same time protecting them on their path.

To the Mind

Kali is an incarnation of the goddess warrior Durga.

She presides over time and the life/death cycle.

Kali represents the tough love of a mother, a destroyer, *shakti* (feminine) energy, and our shadow side all wrapped in a kind benevolence.

Kali, the representative of bold action, appears when we are going through a significant change in our life. During the dark night of the soul, she shows up as strong medicine or tough love to help us navigate the door through which we must pass.

To the Heart

The story of Kali represents transformation and channelling that which is not serving us into something more powerful. She is the goddess to invoke when you need to take revolutionary action in your life. When we are in difficulty or need help, during times of crisis, she appears when we most need her, her tongue blazing red, dressed in wild ragged locks, a necklace of skulls, a skirt of arms, and holding an axe to support and protect us.

This divine devoted mother will shroud you with her primal female power. She is willing us to stare straight into her angry eyes and face our difficulties; if we don't turn to look at our illusions and fears, we will be chased by them instead.

Kali has the power to burn through and reshape our lives' wildfires. We can submit to her burning whatever is not serving us—our stories, our drama, our ways of being, our challenges, and our difficulties.

From the ash, we have the power to rise again, like the phoenix from the flame.

To the Body

❧ *Transform with Kali* ☙

We all have a Kali within us that is ready to rise up when needed. Sometimes we need this fierce love for others, to help them move through their difficulties. Sometimes we need this warrior spirit to arise for us.

May this practice encourage us to offer our rage, our fear, our anxiety to the fire of Kali within so she may absorb it and show us how to channel that energy rightfully.

EGO ERADICATOR

This meditation is from the Kundalini tradition. It is said to boost self-confidence and lift energy. It works well when we have something important to do or when we are lacking confidence and need a boost to remember our divinity. It is a spiritual 'you have got this' dose of medicine.

This meditation uses Breath of Fire, or Kapalabhati, which are short sharp exhales with a belly contraction. The emphasis is on the exhale as the inhale is passive.

Note: This breathing technique is not suited for pregnant women or those with breathing difficulties or blood pressure problems. As with any practice, you should stop if you feel dizzy or unwell.

KALI KRIYA

1. Sit comfortably with your spine upright.

2. Raise your arms up so they are positioned like ten o'clock and two o'clock, about 60 degrees from the ground.

3. Curl your fingers in towards your palms and point your thumbs up.

4. Start with four or five long slow breaths to centre you.

5. Breath of Fire is short sharp exhales with belly contraction, followed by a passive inhale, through your nostrils.

6. After your settling breaths, begin Breath of Fire for one minute, exhaling sharply one or two times every second.

7. When you have completed your cycle, take a long inhale as you bring your thumbs to touch above your head.

8. Exhale your hands by your sides.

9. Repeat two more times.

KALI VINYASA

Goddess pose is sometimes called High Squat or Horse pose. This Goddess vinyasa combines breath and movement with static holds and strength building in the legs.

1. Inhale, straighten your legs and lift your hands to the sky.

2. Exhale, bend your legs into Goddess and bring your hands to your heart. Repeat this movement three times.

3. Inhale, straighten your legs and lift your hands to the sky.

4. Exhale, bend your legs into Goddess and wrap your right arm under your left for Eagle Arms.

5. Inhale, straighten your legs and lift your hands to the sky.

6. Exhale, bend your legs into Goddess and wrap your left arm under your right for Eagle Arms.

7. Inhale, straighten your legs and lift your hands to the sky.

8. Exhale, bend your legs into Goddess and bring your hands out to the sides.

9. Inhale to prepare, exhale, and like a willow tree bow to the right; your right arm will cross in front of your belly and your left arm sway overheard.

10. Inhale to centre, bring your arms out to shoulder height.

11. Exhale, bow to the left, this time your left arm will cross in front and your right arm will go overhead. Inhale to centre. Repeat these movements four or five times on each side.

12. Exhale, place your hands on your thighs.

13. Inhale to prepare.

14. Exhale, drop your right shoulder to your left knee and twist towards your left.

15. Inhale to centre.

16. Exhale, drop your left shoulder to your right knee and twist towards your right.

KALI MUDRA

This powerful mudra is the symbol of the fierce Kali, or Durga, the goddesses that invoke cutting through illusion and obstacles to bring the dark to light. Kali represents the slaying of illusions, the death of the old, and transformation towards higher ways of living.

The left thumb crosses over the right thumb to call upon the feminine qualities of this mudra. It can be performed with the arms straight and overhead, at the heart with the index fingers pointing forwards, or away from the heart with straight arms as if you were holding an axe.

1. Stand in Goddess pose with your feet turned out and a wide stance.

2. Interlace your middle, ring, and little fingers; keep your index fingers pointing forwards like a sword.

3. Cross your left thumb over your right thumb.

4. Inhale, straighten your legs, raise your mudra above your head.

5. Exhale, bend your legs, and chop the mudra between your legs, letting out a loud *Ha* sound.

6. Repeat the chopping five to ten times.

KALI MOON

1. Stand tall in Mountain pose with Kali mudra above your head.

2. Stretch through all sides of your waist.

3. Inhale, squeeze your ears with your arms and look up.

4. Exhale, press strongly into your feet and bow to the right.

5. Inhale to stand.

6. Exhale, bow to your left.

7. Inhale to stand.

8. Squeeze your legs firmly to your midline, press into your feet, and exhale lean back.

KALI FIERCE

1. Come into Fierce (Chair) pose with Kali mudra above your head.

2. Take a breath in and stretch your arms up.

3. Exhale, chop your mudra to the right of your knees.

4. Inhale, lift your mudra back to the sky.

5. Exhale, chop to the left of your knees.

6. Continue with the Kriya for one minute. Stand and absorb in Mountain pose.

KALI BREATHES

Also known as Lion's Breath, this breath relieves tension in the jaw, face, and throat and is a great way to heat up some confidence so you can move through your challenges. This breath can be performed in Down Dog or as below, in a seated posture.

1. Sit on your shins with your knees apart.

2. Place your hands on the floor between your legs, turn your fingers out to the sides or towards your body.

3. Take a long inhalation through both nostrils.

4. Open your mouth as wide as you can, stick out your tongue as if you wanted to touch the tip of your tongue to your chin and let out a long loud *haaaaaa* sound.

5. Repeat three to four times.

Transform with Kali

1   KALI KRIYA

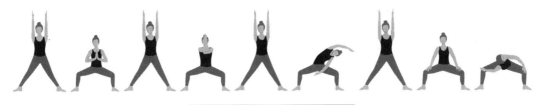

2   KALI VINYASA

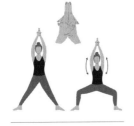

3   KALI MUDRA

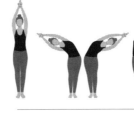

4   KALI MOON

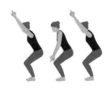

5   KALI FIERCE

6 KALI BREATHES

Teaching Notes

✦ Use mantra to round out the Kali theme.

Beej or bija mantra, meaning seed, are powerful, one syllable sounds that can be chanted alone or as part of longer mantra. When chanted they are said to summon miracles as they work in unseen ways in the universe. When chanted with love and devotion they are said to endow the practitioner with certain qualities or powers.

For protection, power and strength and to dispel fear, repeat the mantra *Om Kreem Kali*, 108 times. Kreem is another word for Kali, to invoke Kali.

✦ Pair Goddess pose with Warrior poses to embody the warrior element of this practice.

✦ Concentrate on longer holds to build strength and fire.

✦ Fire ceremonies or flames give us a physical opportunity to literally burn what we are holding on to. Write down on paper what you want to let go of or transform and throw it to the heat. This theme would work well at the end of a retreat or training.

To Your Life

Kali is the goddess of destruction that makes way for our good. You can call upon her fierce feminine power or shakti to

✦ destroy any habits, attachments, or thoughts that no longer serve you

✦ help you step up to what frightens you

✦ teach you how to say no

✦ shake up any complacency and show you how to invoke change

✦ guide you through vulnerability

✦ release yourself from the bondage of a destructive habit

✦ help you guide others who are faced with the dark night of the soul

✦ unleash your wild feminine spirit

✦ deal with conflict

Place a picture of Kali on your altar. Imagine her qualities of strength, protection, and transformation become part of your dialogue every time you pass or sit with her.

SHIVA THE DANCER

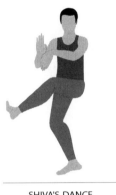

SHIVA'S DANCE

Turn and face the change.
DAVID BOWIE

To the Mind

Si: benevolent

Shiva: the male energy of death and destruction; thought to be one of the originators of yoga or *Adi Guru* ('first yogi').

Shiva is often depicted as the blue-skinned, dreadlocked deity. It is said that his skin is blue because he drank the poison of the world and held it in his throat.

A *jnana* (knowledge or self-study) yogi, he is worshipped by millions at the Kumbh Mela pilgrimage and festival.

Shiva is married to Parvati. Parvati is the goddess of marriage, children, and procreation. She balances his masculinity with her feminine shakti energy. She tames his temper and volatile ways, moving him from the passionate warrior to her serene and tranquil lover.

To the Heart

In this life, there is nothing more certain than change. Many changes or new beginnings have their roots in loss or disruption or sometimes chaos.

Often, we want things to stay the same because in sameness lies safety. Fear and anxiety arise as a by-product of the unknown, so desiring the status quo is natural but also very limiting.

What if we could turn to face the change with grace and see it for what it is: a challenge for our evolution?

The idea of beginnings, maintenance, and endings as represented by Brahma, Vishnu, and Shiva can be found in many aspects of our lives and is obeyed by nature:

+ birth, life, and death

+ the beginning of a yoga class, the central part of the class, and Savasana

+ spring, summer, and autumn/winter

+ the beginning of a relationship, the relationship, and the parting

+ gaining, holding, and letting go

+ the inhale, the pause, and the exhale

+ generate, organise, destroy (g.o.d.)

Nature reminds us of the inherent order of things. That in the worst of its upheavals— severe flooding, earthquakes, and fire—destruction is not always about death; it is there to make way for life.

Shiva represents what needs to be destroyed to create. Without destruction, there is no construction; without loss, there is no gain; without space, there is no room for growth.

Shiva asks us, can you dance through all of life's ups and downs? Can you find bliss amidst the disruption? Can you love the endings as much as the beginnings?

To the Body

⤳ *Shiva* ⤳

This practice prepares the body for Dancer's pose by opening the hamstrings, hip flexors, and shoulders. Incorporate some gentle backbends in your sequence. You can repeat the sequence starting with Dancer's pose.

As with any peak flow sequence, don't be afraid to revisit the peak pose many times, in similar shapes and in the peak form of the pose.

SHIVA'S DANCE

1. Stand on your right leg.

2. Lift your left inner foot off the ground.

3. Turn your left foot towards your right knee.

4. Face your right palm forwards.

5. Turn your left palm down to face your left knee.

AEROPLANE

1. Balance on your right leg.

2. Send your left leg behind you.

3. Bring your arms in line with the sides of your body.

HIGH LUNGE

1. Slowly bend into your right leg.

2. Step your left toes towards the back of the mat.

3. Bend your right leg towards ninety degrees.

4. Take your arms above your head.

WARRIOR TWO

1. Turn your right heel flat.

2. Open your arms out in line with your shoulders.

WIDE LEG FORWARD FOLD

1. Turn both of your feet to face the long edge of the mat.

2. Interlace your hands behind your back.

3. Bow your torso to the floor.

LOW LUNGE

1. Place your hands on the floor.

2. Turn your right foot and torso to the front edge of the mat.

3. Drop your left knee to the ground.

4. Lift your chest and arms to the sky.

5. Bind your arms behind your back.

MONKEY TAIL

1. Bring your forearms to the floor.

2. Sweep your right arm behind you.

3. Kick up your left leg.

4. Bind your left foot with your right hand.

5. Turn your chest to the right.

6. Repeat entire sequence on the other side.

Shiva

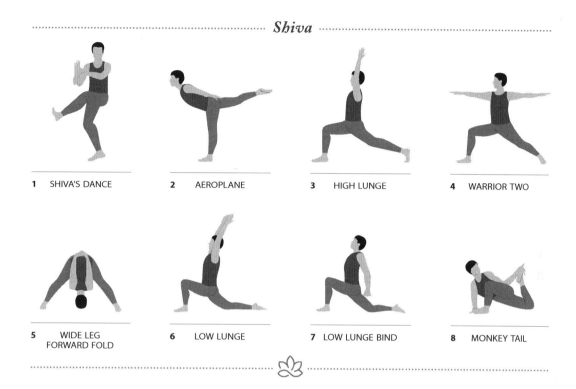

1 SHIVA'S DANCE

2 AEROPLANE

3 HIGH LUNGE

4 WARRIOR TWO

5 WIDE LEG FORWARD FOLD

6 LOW LUNGE

7 LOW LUNGE BIND

8 MONKEY TAIL

Teaching Notes

✦ Shiva is the lord of destruction but his energy is necessary to make way for the creative force of Brahma. Powerful breath techniques such as Bellows Breath—short, sharp, even exhales and inhales—emulate the forceful movement of his prana.

✦ Shiva expresses his divinity through dance (*tandava*). There are two forms of the dance—Ananda Tandava (pictured above), which is Shiva in his purest, most blissful state untouched by the world, and the Rudra Tandava, which is the dance of destruction leading to creation.

✦ The Rudra Tandava dance represents the cycle of birth and death, creation and dissolution. This cycle is embodied in a yoga class—the warm-ups, the peak, and Savasana; the inhales, the holds, and exhales; the pose, the transition, the next pose. Consider the whole class to be a form of Rudra Tandava, leading to Ananda Tandava or Savasana. (See also Vinyasa, the section on transitions.)

✦ Every time we lie down at the end of a class, we get to untangle ourselves from our attachment to the status quo by practising a little death in Savasana pose. Consider inserting Savasana between poses or sets of poses.

✦ Spend time examining the breath mindfully, where it begins in the body, where it is sustained, and what happens at the end of the breath.

✦ Choose poses that encourage joy through diversity; for example, more challenging backbends to express our ability to move through life's difficult circumstances but still retain a 'bliss' feeling.

✦ Sequences that express the qualities of tandava are masculine, dynamic, energetic, creative, free flow expressions, and ecstatic movements.

✦ Shiva is also represented as the Lord of the Dance pose or Natarajasana.

✦ Perform Shiva mudra by turning your left hand palm up at your navel and placing your right fist into your left palm with your thumb pointing up. The left hand represents feminine energy and the thumb of the right hand masculine. Together they also look a little like a flame rising from the ground.

To Your Life

Consider which part of the cycle of life you like; is it beginnings, middles, or ends? What is your view on endings or dissolutions? One of the *kleshas*, or obstacles, on the path to liberation, is *abhinivesha*, which means fear of death, of change, and wanting things to stay the same. By invoking Shiva energy, instead of fearing, we step into the natural flow of life.

Om Namah Shivaya: I bow to Shiva
I offer myself to the light

If you feel stuck in your life, or an end is approaching, chant this transformative mantra 108 times to dissolve and break down old ways of thinking and to give you courage to step into the unknown.

Follow the mantra with Savasana, or Corpse pose. This pose represents death to what has come before, in order to clean the slate for what is to come.

Om Namah Shivaya Gurave
Satchiidananda Murtaye
Nishprapanchaya Shantaya
Niralambaya Tejase
Om[12]

---

[12] *I bow to the Shiva, I bow to all creation | I bow to the teacher within and I open my heart up to this power and grace | I bow to the light within that is never absent and radiates bliss and peace | May this light guide our way leading us towards transformation*

ARJUNA THE WARRIOR

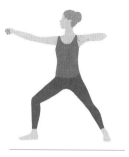

ARCHER WARRIOR

We must be willing to let go of the life we planned so as to have the life that is waiting for us.
JOSEPH CAMPBELL

To the Mind

Vira: hero

Bhadra: friend

Virabhadrasana: Warrior pose

Arjuna, an accomplished warrior with extraordinary powers, is the protagonist in one of the greatest stories from Indian mythology. Known as the love song to the divine, the *Bhagavad Gita* is a conversation between Arjuna and his beloved Krishna, who metaphorically is his higher self, his guide, and god. The story is symbolic of the inner struggles we must face every day. The dialogue Arjuna has with Krishna is a conversation we must have with ourselves—a call and response to our higher self.

THE BHAGAVAD GITA

The *Gita* is part of a larger text known as the *Mahabharata*.

In the story, Krishna teaches three paths of yoga:

+ karma yoga: the yoga of action or to work without attachment to the results

+ jnana yoga: the path of knowledge, through self-study, contemplation, and meditation

+ bhakti yoga: the path of devotion to god/love

The story begins at the start of a cataclysmic battle. Just before the battle is about to start, Arjuna asks his friend Krishna, the charioteer, to take him to the line so he can observe what is to play out. When he arrives, he sees his friends, teachers, and family on both sides.

On one side of the field stand the good and virtuous Pandava brothers, who fight to serve all and are devoted to Krishna and the good of man. On the other side are the disreputable Kauravas, motivated by greed and known for their ignorance and wrongdoings. Arjuna knows the soldiers from both sides.

Overwhelmed, Arjuna realises he will have to kill his friends and relatives, and in his despair, his heart cracks wide open.

Krishna counsels him, 'Arjuna! Get up. This is not the time for you to give in. Sitting on the fence is not an option. You are a warrior of the highest, you have encountered much more than this. Get up and take aim; rise to meet your challenges. You have the capacity and skills. Do your duty. I will give you some options from the path of yoga, and once you understand them, you will be able to act. However, Arjuna, in the end, you must do as you please; you must live your life and make your own choices.'

Don't ask yourself what the world needs. Ask yourself what makes you come alive, and do that, because what the world needs is people who have come alive.

HOWARD THURMAN

Remember, when you say yes to one thing you say no to another. The best choice will be the one that comes from the conversation with your higher self and aligns with your values.

Do your best and let go of the results of your actions. All you can do is your job, so do it with love, to the best of your ability. You are not powerful enough to determine the outcome.

To the Heart

You are as unique as the life line on your hand
You came here with a purpose
A symphony in your soul and a song to sing
Your composition is so valuable
Others have seen it in you, and now it's your turn

Take a look!
When you know your duty
You will become radiantly alive
And all your days will be harmonious.

DHARMA

Deep within the cocoon of our being lies our soul's mandate, our purpose for embodiment. Each of us has a unique gift or reason for being here—our *dharma*—and our duty is to uncover this purpose. When you entered this world, you made a contract with your soul to write the unwritten composition of your heart.

Do something you love; that is your dharma.

The *Gita* reminds us that it is better to live out our dharma poorly than to carry out another's well.

The universe is asking you to step up, to not leave before singing the unsung, to bring what you value and gift it to the world.

To determine our true nature or calling, we must be prepared to look and listen within. When we define our purpose for being on this earth, we set our legacy in motion. By following our true nature, and the dream of our heart with love, it becomes an offering, a service for the higher good.

Dharma is

+ to do something that you love

+ to live following your higher values and purpose

+ to unveil the mission of your soul

We have personal dharma, but there is also a collective one. Our calling should bind or glue us to the more extensive web of life that supports the natural intelligence of the greater whole.

MEDITATION—EMBRACING YOUR DHARMA

Sit quietly and comfortably.
Feel the shape of your body and where your body touches the floor.
Feel the clothes on your skin and the skin on your bones.

Feel into the entire shape of your container.

Now dive deeper and feel inside the vault of your heart.

Feel the pulse of life surge within, your leading light, the place you call your soul or spirit or energy body.

Like a star, this energy is unique to you. This part signed up for your journey.

You arrived here for a reason, and your purpose lies in the uniqueness and gifts you bring to this world.

May you live a life appreciating your talents and may your choices empower and impel you to live a dharma-filled day.

To the Body

❥ *Meet the Warriors* ❦

The warrior Virabhadra was born from a family quarrel.

Daksha, Shiva's father-in-law, was holding a party, but he refused entry to Shiva in order to protect his daughter, Sati, from this dreadlocked wild man. Sati was so distraught she threw herself onto the bonfire. In retaliation, Shiva tore out his hair and threw it to the ground, and *Virabhadrasana One*, or Warrior One, was born.

This complex pose with all its twists and bends will reveal to you your physical blind spots and ask you to rise above your limitations. Warrior One was born out of chaos, jealousy, and destruction. When we stand in the pose, we are being asked to face our obstacles and to throw into the fire whatever stands between us and truth.

Virabhadra One: Shiva arises from the ground with his sword clasped above his head.
Virabhadra Two: Shiva stands in preparation for battle.
Virabhadra Three: Shiva springs into action and takes off the head of Sati's father.

Challenge your fear, embrace your strength, and choose your battles in strong standing Warrior poses.

THE DANCE OF THE WARRIOR
From Down Dog

1. Crescent Lunge. Step your left leg towards your right hand. Lift your torso away from the floor and reach your arms for the sky.
2. Reverse Crescent Lunge. Slide your right hand down the back of your right thigh and arch your left arm towards the back of your mat.
3. Revolved Crescent Lunge variation. Bring your arms back skywards to Crescent Lunge. Open your arms to the long, left side of your mat at shoulder height.
4. Revolved Crescent Lunge. Join your palms together, lean your torso forwards, and hook your right elbow over your bent left leg.
5. Warrior Two. Swing your torso up and around to face the long right edge of the mat. Turn your right foot flat; open your arms to shoulder height.
6. Reverse Warrior Two. Slide your right hand down your right thigh, and arch your left arm and torso towards the back of the mat.

BOW TO THE WARRIOR WITHIN
From Down Dog

1. Warrior One. Step your right leg towards your right hand. Turn your back foot flat. Lift your torso away from the floor and reach your arms for the sky.
2. Warrior One Bind. Interlace your fingers behind your back.
3. Humble Warrior. Bow inside of your right leg or rest your torso on your leg.

4. Archer Warrior. Lift your torso back up so your shoulders are stacked over your hips. Undo your bind. Turn your back foot so the toes face the long edge of the mat and come into Warrior Two with your arms at shoulder height and your palms facing the long edge of the mat. Make fists with both hands. Bend your back arm and place your fist on your chest. Take aim.
5. Archer Warrior Reverse. Arch your right arm and torso towards the back of the mat.

COURAGEOUS WARRIOR
From Down Dog

1. Warrior Two. Step your right leg towards your right hand. Lift your torso up and stack your shoulders over your hips. Bring your arms to shoulder height.
2. Warrior Two variation. Bring both of your arms overhead. Lean your body towards the right. Engage your core.
3. Reverse Warrior. Slide your left hand down your left thigh; arch your right arm and torso towards the back of the mat.
4. Side Angle. Bring your torso upright to Warrior Two position. Transition to Side Angle by placing your right forearm on your right thigh and reaching your left arm to the sky or across your ear to the front of the mat.
5. Runners Lunge. Turn your torso and frame your right leg by placing both hands on either side of your foot. Swivel your back heel up to the sky.

WARRIOR TAKES AIM

From Down Dog

1. Crescent Lunge. Step your left leg towards your left hand. Lift your torso and raise your arms to the sky.

2. Warrior Three. Lean your torso and arms forwards, then lift your back foot off the floor so your entire body starts to make a giant 'T' shape.

3. Standing Splits. Hinge at the hips and place your hands on the floor or blocks on either side of your left foot.

4. Seated Twist. Bend your left knee and bring your bent right leg to the back of your front leg. Slowly slide your back leg down to the floor. Turn your torso to the left and hook your right elbow over your left knee.

Meet the Warriors

THE DANCE OF THE WARRIOR

1 CRESCENT LUNGE 2 REVERSE CRESCENT LUNGE 3 REVOLVED CRESCENT LUNGE VARIATION 4 REVOLVED CRESCENT LUNGE 5 WARRIOR TWO 6 REVERSE WARRIOR TWO

BOW TO THE WARRIOR WITHIN

1 WARRIOR ONE 2 WARRIOR ONE BIND 3 HUMBLE WARRIOR 4 ARCHER WARRIOR 5 ARCHER WARRIOR REVERSE

COURAGEOUS WARRIOR

1 WARRIOR TWO 2 WARRIOR ONE VARIATION 3 REVERSE WARRIOR 4 SIDE ANGLE 5 RUNNER'S LUNGE

WARRIOR TAKES AIM

1 CRESCENT WARRIOR 2 WARRIOR THREE 3 STANDING SPLITS 4 SEATED TWIST

Teaching Notes

In the Warrior poses, can you find the qualities of a warrior?

+ Energy without aggression

+ Strong but open-hearted

+ A balance of will and surrender

+ Fearlessness and gentleness. The body of a warrior, the heart of a monk.

+ Variations include Humble Warrior, Down Dog Warrior, Reverse Crescent Warrior, Reverse Warrior Two, and Goddess pose.

+ Blocks will support Warrior Three variation and Hero pose.

+ Use Hero pose and her variations to build your theme. (See also Vajrasana in Opening Poses.) Hero pose can bring up physical restrictions for students, which plays nicely into the theme of the Warrior: facing your difficulties and choosing your battles.

+ Longer holds in Warrior poses will build strength and courage. Try ten breath counts to challenge the status quo.

+ You could theme your class around seated or standing Archer's pose as a peak pose.

+ Arjuna was an accomplished archer. Poses that emulate the archer's bow, such as Bow pose and variations, tie in with the theme.

+ 'Meet the Warriors' is creative play on the classic Warrior poses. You can add a vinyasa after each set, (High Plank, Low Plank, Up Dog, Down Dog.) You can do all the sets or choose to do one and repeat it. Start on either the left or the right side and repeat on the other side.

To Your Life

THE WARRIOR HEART

Each day sees a new challenge and many little battles. To live fearlessly, we must hold the qualities of a warrior at our heart: steadiness, stability, and courage.

The challenges warriors face are opportunities to become a little more resilient, a little more robust. Enter your challenges being willing to fight the good fight but willing to let go of the results.

Choose what is worth fighting for in life.

ON SURRENDER

To surrender is to step away from control and micromanagement of our life. When we accept that there is a greater good that governs our life force we lean into a more easeful life.

ON TAKING SIDES

You will often be pulled from the centre. Like a master chess player, widen your vision to see the bigger picture from all angles, and make your choices from this bird's eye view. Instead of choosing sides, choose to remain true to your core values, to your centre.

CHOOSE LOVE OVER FEAR

The final message of the *Gita* is to choose love and devotion. Krishna's last words are 'to think of me always,' a reminder to give our love freely and to accept the love that comes our way. Choosing to love in this way dispels our fear.

If you feel challenged, stuck, unsure, fearful, or hidden, remember the qualities of the warrior: fearless and on a mission of love and the love of Krishna.

SUTRA STITCHES

Your vision will become clear only when you can look into your own heart.
Who looks outside, dream; who looks inside, awakens.

CARL JUNG

In this section we weave the various styles and approaches of yoga into the heart of the Sutras.

Often, when we first start yoga, we arrive in our physical body wanting to alleviate an ache or to soften tightness. Maybe we have been cajoled into attending a class by a friend, or we have been prescribed 'yoga' to help us heal.

So we show up, unroll our mat, and move our bodies. The body, with its hidden intelligence, will respond lovingly to the attention we have given it, and other things will start to unfold.

We may find we become more limber, we learn to breathe fully again, and we bathe in the sweet glow of Savasana. Sooner or later, if we are diligent, an enquiry will arise. As we start to enter into a more personal relationship with ourselves, we may begin to peek beyond the physicality and dive into the fuller picture of this age-old practice.

The field of yoga is vast. Once you open one door, it becomes like a hall of mirrors, so knowing which way to go can be daunting. At times you may be swallowed whole by its enormity or wade in uncertainty, but if the intention is there to know more about yourself, you will return again and again.

The philosophy of the ages as codified by Patanjali in the *Yoga Sūtra* is an excellent place to start with self-enquiry. The sutras urge you to be a scientist of self-discovery.

The *Yoga Sūtra* lays out ten principles to incorporate into your practice, known as the *yamas* and *niyamas*. They are a global and relatable map to help us navigate our world. This compass of human nature will help direct our study, and in doing so, we will start to challenge some of our ideas and our ways of living.

When we take time to consider how the teachings relate to our own lives, when we look at our ethics and core values, we become the stewards of change. To deepen our practice means a vote for ourselves. When we cease to be the placeholders of our life, we take a courageous step to invite change and challenge the status quo.

The musk deer spends its entire life searching for the source of an alluring perfume,
never to learn that it arises from itself.

We can choose to wander without question like the musk deer, or we can examine how the teachings relate to our lives and divorce ourselves from the idea that happiness, answers, love, and contentment lie outside of us.

The yoga sutras

Long considered the heart of the yoga practice, the sutras are a framework for self-enquiry that carries encoded messages describing yoga. The *Yoga Sūtras* is a rule book for how to live a life that is less stressful, more meaningful, and that connects you to something more significant that you may not have known existed.

Written around two thousand years ago, the sutras—which means 'stitches'—are attributed to the sage Patanjali, who may have been a scientist, a philosopher, a group of people, or one person. Patanjali took the teachings that had been shared orally through the years and codified them into 196 threads or stitches, explaining what yoga is and how it can be achieved.

The stitches are ordered into four chapters, and each one carries the resonance of the one before, turning the wisdom into a delicate cloth ready to be unravelled by the seeker. The meanings of the passages are infused into the Sanskrit language; like a concentrate they are so distilled that to decode them means to sit with them in our heart until we can breathe life into them.

The sutras were written for an Eastern mind. Eastern practitioners of yoga already had an understanding of the body/mind/nature connection, of spirituality, and ideas about the soul or consciousness.

The Western mind is not so often guided by spirituality. To make these teachings come alive just as they were two thousand years ago, they need to be understood from a Western viewpoint. How can I, as a teacher or practitioner, take the essence of these teachings and use them in my life? It is from this questioning that many of the texts you read today arose—personal interpretations and commentaries of these terse statements.

They explain what happens on the inside, in your mind, emotions, and body, when you do the practice of yoga. They are tools for us to alleviate our suffering.

There are 196 verses divided into four chapters, or 'padas' (feet).

1. *Samadhi Pada* defines what yoga is, or the purpose of yoga.

2. *Sadhana Pada* describes yoga philosophy, the eightfold path of yoga (*ashtanga*), and *kriya* yoga.

3. *Vibhuti Pada* explains the benefits of yoga and the supernatural powers you can gain from practising yoga.

4. *Kaivalya Pada* defines liberation, samadhi, or freedom.

KRIYA YOGA

Kriya yoga as defined by Patanjali is three actions you can take to remove any obstacles that are in the way of obtaining stillness of the mind. These are tapas or discipline, svadhyaya or self-study, and ishvara pranidhana or surrender to a higher power.

May the teachings of the sutras download into our spiritual hearts and minds as we continue on our path towards awakening.

YAMAS/NIYAMAS

The ashtanga principles teach us that to be at peace in life, we must turn our focus towards

+ our relationships with others and the environment (*yama*)

+ our relationship with our self (*niyama*)

+ our body (*asana*)

+ our breath and energy (*pranayama*)

+ our senses (*pratyahara*)

+ our mind (*dharana* and *dhyana*)

Doing so ultimately leads to *samadhi* (liberation). This tree of suggestions about how to live our life free from suffering offers simple, climbable steps we can take each day to walk towards harmony. Each step we take reveals another step or richer layer, taking us closer to balance and peace.

Patanjali lists the yamas and niyamas as skilful ways to get us closer to the state of yoga, which he defines as the stilling of the mind. When the mind stills, we can understand the true nature of our existence.

YAMA

You are the peaceful warrior.

You touch others with kindness, truth, honesty, generosity, and loyalty.

NIYAMA

Your life is your teacher.

The relationship you have with yourself is the most potent one you will ever have.

ASANA

You are a disciple of your body home.

Make contact with the shape of your body. Feel the liaison of your body with all life.

PRANAYAMA

You are a master of your breath.

Drop into the sound of your breath. Turn up the volume until it floods your entire being.

DHARANA-DHYANA-SAMADHI

Water to river to ocean

Concentration to flow to oneness

You are the caretaker, the partner, the guide, and the teacher of the entire universe, which is you.

May this be the sweetest love story of your life.

YAMAS

The first step on the ladder suggests practices to moderate our behaviour so our actions, words, and deeds have a positive impact on all our relationships, including those with the environment.

There are many translations and definitions for the first limb, including

+ bridle or rein: the reins allow the rider (the mind) to direct the horse (the instinct) where it needs to go

+ restrain, subdue, or control our behaviour

+ be nice to others

+ living codes of conduct

+ moral guidelines

+ guidelines for showing our respect for others and the environment

+ the 'do nots'

+ ethical precepts

+ the avoidances on the path

There are five yamas in Patanjali's *Yoga Sūtra*:

• ahimsa
• satya
• asteya
• brahmacharya
• aparigraha

The following section looks at these five principles in more detail and gives suggestions, practices, and ideas about bringing the yamas into modern day life.

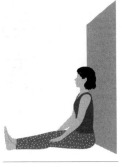

AHIMSA

AHIMSA

To hurt others is to hurt oneself.
To hurt oneself is to hurt others.

UNKNOWN

To the Mind

A: against or not

Himsa: harm, injustice, or cruelty

Ahimsa: do no harm

Ahimsa is the basic act of being kind to yourself and to others in what you say, do, think, eat, buy, take in. Ahimsa is summed up beautifully by Jon Kabat Zinn in his book *Wherever You Go There You Are*: 'Why not try to live to cause as little damage and suffering as possible?'

To the Heart

Ahimsa shows up under different names in many traditions. The first principle of Buddhist philosophy is to see the inner nobility and beauty of all human beings. For Gandhi, ahimsa was his peaceful 'weapon' that he used to overcome conflict, racism, and greed in his fight for justice. Jainism centres its faith around the principle of kindness with the belief that to hurt any living thing is to hurt themselves. Jains lovingly sweep the streets before they walk in the hope not to harm a single bug with their feet. The first principle of medical practitioners and the first most important yama from Patanjali's *Yoga Sūtra* is ahimsa: do no harm.

Einstein tells us one of the most important choices we will ever have to make is whether to believe that the world is a friendly place or not. If we think it is, then we will see more love around us, give and forgive, be kind, and support others. If we think the world is unkind, our energy will be put into building walls and creating separation to protect ourselves from being hurt or harmed.

Like a Russian nesting doll, kindness has many layers. We start with the gross actions of direct service, helping, comforting, listening, and spending time with a lonely soul. Sooner or later, like all the sutras, another layer will bubble to the surface and we will start to apply the lessons to our thoughts and our words.

Ahimsa asks that we say and think kind-hearted things to others and ourselves. Our words are our most important tool for practising this tenet.

The outer critic reflects the inner criticism.
The outer judge reflects inner judgements.
What you say about others says a lot about yourself.

Everything that we do, say, and think has an outwards and inwards reaction.

The litmus test for kindness is simple.

Ask yourself: how does this thought, word, or action feel?

And for those you love: what is the kindest action, word, or thought I can give to you right now?

Feel the answers leading you to higher ground.

To the Body

⭑ *Wall of Kindness* ⭑

When we stake a tomato plant, we are saying, here, take this support as a reminder of what you can do, or how tall you can grow with a little help.

Listening, attention, nurturing, and serving are all ways we can offer our support and kindness to promote growth and healing and to help those we love to expand.

This practice uses the wall as support, not separation, as something to lean into, and a reminder that someone has your back.

May this practice remind you the world is indeed a friendly, kind, and supportive place.

Turn the mat with the short edge to the wall.

WALL BREATHING

1. Sit with your back to the wall.
2. As you lean in, start to take long slow breaths.
3. Feel your breath in the back of your body.

SHOULDER STRETCH

1. Stand about one arm's length away from the wall.
2. Place your forearms on the wall.
3. Clasp your hands.
4. Lean your upper body towards the wall.

WALL CHAIR

1. Stand with your back to the wall and your feet 30 centimetres away from the wall.
2. Bend your knees and lift your hands up above your head.
3. Rest your back on the wall.
4. Stay for a few breaths.

CAT-COW

1. From Wall Chair, lean forwards and place your hands on your thighs.
2. Keep your sit bones on the wall.
3. Inhale, arch the spine as you press your chest forwards.
4. Exhale, curl the spine as you draw your navel into your backbone.

FORWARD FOLD

1. From Cat-Cow, release your spine to bow over your legs.
2. Place your hands on the ground or blocks.
3. Keep your sit bones pressed into the wall.
4. Hold this for a few breaths.
5. Now turn around and fold over; this time press your upper back gently into the wall.

THREE-LEGGED DOG

1. Walk your hands forwards on your mat into Down Dog.
2. Place your feet with your heels up the wall and your toes on the ground.
3. Lift your right leg into the air and press your foot into the wall.
4. Stay here for a few breaths.

CRESCENT LUNGE CLOSED TWIST

1. From Three-Legged Dog, step your right foot forwards into a lunge; keep your left heel up the wall and toes near the skirting board.
2. Lift your arms above your head.
3. Twist; open your arms to the right.
4. Place your right hand on the wall and press into the wall as you twist.

5. Repeat Three-Legged Dog and Crescent Lunge on the left side.

WILLOW TREE

1. Stand with your left side to the wall. You should be one arm's distance away.
2. Place your left hand on the wall.
3. Bring your left leg up into Tree pose.
4. Sweep your right arm over your head to touch the wall on the left side.
5. Your left arm will bend slightly.
6. Repeat on the other side.

COBRA

1. Lie on the floor, stomach-down, with your head touching the wall.
2. Place your hands on the wall a little wider than shoulder-width apart.
3. Lift your chest as you press into the wall.

SEATED TWIST

1. Sit on the floor with your legs crossed.
2. Check you are about one arm's length from the wall.
3. Turn your body to the left and place your left hand on the wall.
4. Place your right hand on your left knee.
5. Repeat on the other side.

Wall of Kindness

| 1 WALL BREATHING | 2 SHOULDER STRETCH | 3 WALL CHAIR | 4 CAT-COW | 5 FORWARD FOLD |

| 6 THREE-LEGGED DOG | 7 CRESCENT LUNGE CLOSED TWIST | 8 WILLOW TREE | 9 COBRA | 10 SEATED TWIST |

Teaching Notes

+ Walls help with grounding, stability, balance and support. So, if any of these are your themes consider doing one or two wall poses in your class.

+ The wall acts as a prop to assist beginners.

+ Wall yoga gives students a different perspective on familiar poses.

+ Walls help with proprioception, knowing where their body is in space, as it creates a boundary.

+ If you plan to teach one or two wall poses, instruct students to set their mats up near the wall before the class starts.

+ If teaching yin, base your sequence around the wall with poses such as Legs up the Wall, Dangling with your seat against the wall, Wide Leg Straddle with your legs on the wall.

To Your Life

As your practice deepens, you may want to consider what you purchase, think, and do on a daily basis.

WHAT YOU PURCHASE

This week, consider something you buy regularly. The action of ahimsa runs deeply alongside our relationship to the planet. With your next purchase, take time to appreciate the hands that brought this to you. Maybe it's at the supermarket checkout where you take time to thank the person who served you, or perhaps you take some time to silently thank the chain of workers that, without being seen, helped bring the food to your plate.

Support manufacturers that operate under the principle of ahimsa by how they treat the environment and their workers.

WHAT YOU DO

Consider your small daily actions as mini-demonstrations of kindness.

+ pick up some rubbish

+ forgive someone

+ consider if gossiping about someone makes you feel good in the long term

+ leave a kind note for someone

✦ do something without asking or expecting thanks

✦ look at yourself in the mirror and recognise something beautiful about yourself

✦ consider vegetarianism or veganism for a meal, a day, a week

WHAT YOU THINK

The Three Gates

Sufism tells us that written, spoken, or internal words must pass through three gates if we are to become liberated from our fear, our judging, and our harsh inner voice:

Is it true?

Is it kind?

Is it necessary?

Sit quietly. Reflect on or journal about a consistent, unloving thought that you have about yourself.

I am…

I wish I were…

I'm not…

I'm always…

If only…

I can't…

When we have an internal dialogue, we should ask: is it true, is it kind, is it useful? Is the silent talk freeing us and taking us to higher places, or is it holding us back from living a life that is compassionate, gentle, and loving towards our self?

We can't stop our thoughts; they are secreted from the brain to protect us, to help us avoid pain. What we can do is question their validity, to be on guard when we feel we are entering dangerous territory, to learn humility when we stumble over our internal words and to always, always, be kind.

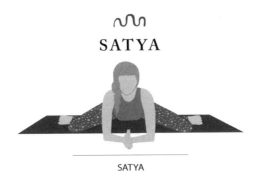

SATYA

SATYA

The truth shall set you free.

JOHN 8:32

To the Mind

Sat: truth or essence

Satsang: true company

Satyagraha: holding on to the truth

Asat: untruth

Satya has many definitions—honesty, genuine, authenticity, being truthful with ourselves and with others, having true intentions, having integrity, not misleading others or deceiving others (or ourselves), or not obscuring the truth.

Satchidananda: pure and blissful. When you strip away all that is not your 'essential' self, the untruths, you find yourself in a state of bliss.

Satyagraha: translates roughly as truth-force or the force that is generated through adherence to truth. In history, satyagraha was a movement started by Gandhi in the peaceful fight to win the battle for India's independence.

Sat Nam: Truth is my identity, true name

Sat Nam is one of the most used mantras in the Kundalini tradition. It is said that when we chant it, the energy 'I am truth' permeates deep into our being. The vibration of the mantra will break your heart open, and you will realise your purpose for this life. When we take action towards our legacy or reason for being here, we demonstrate integrity. Integrity comes from the root 'to make whole again,' to unite yourself with your true self.

To the Heart

The greatest lies we believe are the ones we tell ourselves.

THE STORIES WE TELL

At ground level, satya is being honest and not lying or covering over the truth. Lying is an outer reflection of our internal instability and fears. When we lie, we are glossing over or hiding behind our words for some self-serving purpose.

Being honest with someone is not always practising satya. When we openly counsel others without them asking, tell others what we 'think,' give someone an 'honest' opinion on the way they act, dress, or behave, we are too raw. Satya follows ahimsa, so we always remember that sometimes to be kind is to omit the 'truth'.

Deeper below the everyday workings of our words lie our innermost beliefs, values, and stories shaped by our upbringing, our genetics, and our collective experiences. We were unwittingly taught by our caregivers to look at ourselves and life in a certain way. Lodged deeply in our psyche, the words become the story and our reality.

Any story is a container that limits who we are. A box has six sides. If we only look at one side of the box, we can't see the other sides. The side we look at is the one that is 'true', but it is just one perspective. If we step back, we may see that each of the sides has a story, and the truth will unlock them and open the container up.

To the Body

❧ *Truthful alternatives* ☙

Yin yoga, as with all yoga practices, is one where you meet your body where it is at today. When we fine-tune our senses and converse with our inner world, we know in which direction to point our practice.

The poses chosen here are more on the challenging side. This practice requires you to be honest about what variation of the posture you take. Two versions of each pose are given; the first pose is considered 'milder.'

INTENTION SETTING

What do you need from your practice today? Try to discern what you think you want from what you truly need. If what you truly need is to lie down for an hour in Savasana, be courageous enough to do that. If it is to come out of the pose, be brave and either lie down or try a different variation.

Remember, it takes more energy to resist our truths then to follow them, even if it does create initial friction.

NODDING BREATH—SAYING 'YES' TO YOU

1. Sit comfortably, lengthen your spine, and lift and expand through your chest.

2. Take a cleansing breath in for a count of eight, then release your breath slowly for a count of eight.

3. Add a hold at the top: inhale for a count of eight, hold for a count of four, exhale for a count of eight.

4. Now, add a nodding movement of the head and a slight lift of the sternum as you bring your chin to your chest:

5. Start with your chin close to your chest.

6. As you inhale for eight, lift your chin to be parallel with the floor.

7. Hold here for four counts. Lift your sternum a little and lengthen through the back of your skull.

8. Exhale for eight counts as you nod your head back towards your chest.

9. Repeat, inhale for a count of eight as you lift your chin, hold for four, exhale for a count of eight as you drop your head.

10. Repeat for five more rounds. Each round is a nod to yourself, your life, and a recognition that you are on the right path.

TOE SQUAT

Option one: Toes tucked under in Child's pose.

Option two: Toes tucked under with your chest and head stacked over your heels.

DRAGON SPLITS

Option one: Lie on your belly and spread your left leg out to the left on the floor. Your right leg will point back directly from your right hip.

Option two: Lunge your left leg forwards and drop your right knee to the ground. Straighten your left leg as much as possible.

SQUARE POSE

Option one: Bring your left leg shin in line with the front of the mat. Bring your right leg at right angles with your shin in line with the side of the mat. Both legs are at around 90 degrees.

Option two: From a seated position, bend your left leg and place the shin parallel to the front of the mat. Stack your right leg shin on top of your left shin.

SADDLE

Begin lying on your back.

Option one: Bend your knees and place your feet to the edges of the mat. Drop your knees over to the left side. Repeat to the right.

Option two: Sit on to your calves or between your calves. Slowly lower your back to the floor.

FROG

Option one: Lying on your back, place your sit bones against a wall. Place your legs on the wall and separate them into a 'v' shape.

Option two: From kneeling, separate your knees wide to the sides of the mat. Place your forearms on the floor or a block.

SNAIL

Option one: From a seated posture, lengthen your legs forwards and bow over your legs.

Option two: Lie on your back, roll your pelvis and legs up and to the floor behind you. Support your back with your hands if needed.

Truthful Alternatives

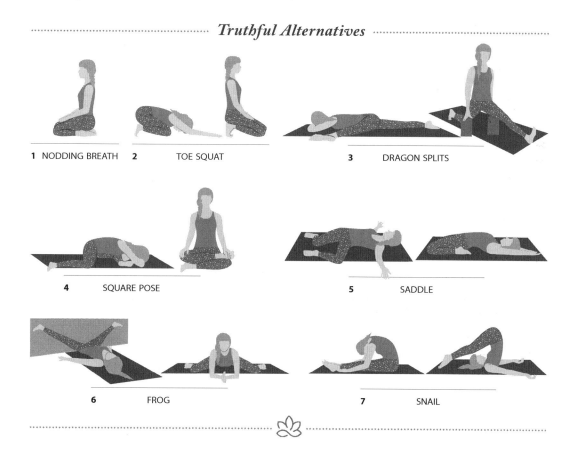

1 NODDING BREATH   2   TOE SQUAT

3   DRAGON SPLITS

4   SQUARE POSE

5   SADDLE

6   FROG

7   SNAIL

Teaching Notes

✦ Demonstrate both poses.

Remind students

✦ the body never lies

✦ be honest with where your body and mind are today

✦ listen to your body; it will show you the way

✦ take as many props as you need

✦ to be true to yourself and the practice is to be present

To Your Life

To thine own self be true.

SHAKESPEARE

Satya is the kernel of truth in our hearts that expresses itself through our thoughts, words, and actions.

This week, as you practise off the mat, consider the little ways in which you can manipulate the truth. Examine every action or inaction, every thought or thoughts you don't want to have. Are these things bringing you closer to what is true for you?

Do you

✦ lie to gain approval or to cover a fear?

✦ make excuses? Excuses are a form of dishonesty. With love and compassion, can you say what you mean or want instead? To recognise who we are and what we want from this life requires a molecule of courage.

✦ say yes or no to things when you should state the opposite? When we agree to something for the wrong reasons, we are not practising satya.

✦ project an outward composure to hide your internal reality? Consider ways to kindly and compassionately express to others what you feel.

Other ideas:

+ During meditation, ask for guidance from your higher self.

+ Consider how it feels when you speak an untruth.

+ To have integrity, you must first know your values. What are your moral codes for life?

+ Be authentic. Observe your desire to copy others. Imitation is not always the highest form of flattery; it can be an expression of inauthenticity.

+ Take time to consider the effects of what you say.

+ Change your language to 'I feel sadness' or 'there is sadness in me' as opposed to 'I am sad.' This rewording helps us remember to not identify with passing (untrue, unreal, temporary) states.

+ Take time to work out how you want to live in the world, to earn and serve.

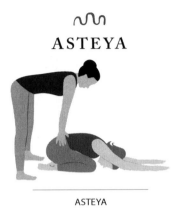

ASTEYA

ASTEYA

Comparison is the thief of joy.
THEODORE ROOSEVELT

To the Mind

A: not
steya: to steal

Asteya, the Sanskrit word for not stealing, includes the physical act of taking as well as the *intention* to take what is not rightfully ours.

Taking what is not freely offered has so many grey and subtle tones. The more delicate layers of asteya may not be so obvious. Asteya covers all the ways we can 'steal' from others and the planet, including words, time, ideas, and behaviours. It also covers the action of stealing from yourself. For when you take from another, you are unwittingly subtracting something from yourself.

To the Heart

EMOTIONAL ROBBERY
Our dramas, problems, and messes are ours. When we 'dump' them unsolicited onto another, we drain that person's emotional bank balance.

PEACE STEALER
Peace can be given and taken. Taking away someone's peace of mind, heart, or physical peace is spiritually and energetically draining.

UN-PLAGIARISE YOUR LIFE

It's relatively easy to look at someone's life, to how they are living, and want to emulate that. However, when we copy others' words or ideas without giving them credit, or try to cut and paste another's life into our own, we are, in a sense, stealing.

TIME VAMPIRE

Keeping others waiting or always being late yourself, taking up someone's time through speech, are ways we may cut into another's precious time.

ENVIRONMENTAL BANDIT

There is plenty to go around in the ever-generous world. Taking more than you need from the environment, wasting the world's precious resources, or stockpiling, all diminish shared resources to the point of depletion.

PRANA DRAINER

Unwise use of your energy, overcommitting, or working yourself to the bone is a withdrawal from the energetic bank balance. When we go into the red, we steal from our health.

Steya is a band-aid we use to cover the feelings of lack.

When we take just what we need, we feed ourselves so we can be of service to others.

When we take just what we need, we reserve the right for others to have their share.

When we take just what we need, we respect the finite nature of the world's resources.

When we take just what we need, we live in psychological abundance and desire falls away.

Through giving back, we replenish what we have subtracted.

To the Body

❧ *Partner Yoga* ❧

When we practice yoga in partnership, we honour the act of sharing. Sharing is an antidote to taking. Partner yoga requires us to be fully in touch with the needs of others, to be in communication, to give and take, and to be energetically and physically supportive of our partner. Partner poses establish the spirit of trust, which is another keystone of asteya.

When we work in teams, we remember that life and yoga is a relationship.

BACK BREATHING

1. Sit in Easy Seat.
2. Rest your back against your partner's back.
3. Breathe in and out and feel the rise and fall of your partner's breath.

EASY SEAT TWIST

1. From Back Breathing, turn your torso to the right.
2. Place your left hand on your right knee.
3. Place your right hand on your partner's left knee.
4. Your partner does the opposite.
5. Repeat on the other side.

LATERAL LEAN

1. From Easy Seat, press softly into your partner's back.
2. Both partners raise your arms above your head.
3. Hold on to your partner's left hand with your left hand.
4. Bow to your right.
5. Repeat on the other side.

CHAIR COBRA

1. Invite your partner to lie on the floor with their arms behind them.
2. Step to the feet of your partner and pick up their wrists or hands.
3. Bend your knees and slowly lift your partner's chest off the ground.

DOG CHILD

1. Invite your partner into Child's pose.
2. Stand at your partner's head.
3. Ask your partner to hold your ankles.

4. Fold Forward and press your partner's sacrum back and down.

CHAIR TWIST

1. Stand a metre away from your partner and face them.
2. Both partners bend at the knees and sink into Chair pose.
3. Hold out your right hand and grasp your partner's left hand.
4. Lean back slightly.
5. Turn to your left.
6. Open your left hand behind you.
7. Repeat on the other side.

CHAIR POSE

1. Turn back-to-back.
2. Press your backs to each other and lean in.
3. Interlace your arms with your partner's.
4. Bend your knees and sit into Chair pose.
5. Stay for five breaths.

STANDING SHOULDER OPENER

1. Stand to face your partner, about a metre apart.
2. Hold your partner's wrists.
3. Both partners fold at the hips to make an 'L' shape.

WIDE LEG STRADDLE

1. Both partners sit facing each other.
2. Take your legs out wide.
3. Connect the soles of your feet with the soles of your partner's feet.
4. Hold your partner's hands.
5. Gently lean back; your partner will lean forwards.

6. Stay for a few breaths.

7. Switch so that you lean forwards and your partner leans back.

DOUBLE DANCER

1. Stand and face your partner.

2. Join your right palms together.

3. Press slightly into your partner as you grasp your left ankle.

4. Arch your left leg up behind you.

5. Imitate Baby Cobra in your upper back.

6. Repeat on the other side.

Partner Yoga

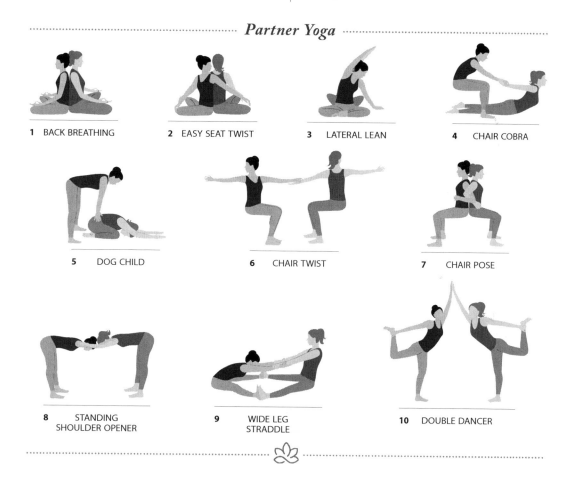

1 BACK BREATHING

2 EASY SEAT TWIST

3 LATERAL LEAN

4 CHAIR COBRA

5 DOG CHILD

6 CHAIR TWIST

7 CHAIR POSE

8 STANDING SHOULDER OPENER

9 WIDE LEG STRADDLE

10 DOUBLE DANCER

Teaching Notes

✦ If someone is unwilling or unable to join in, you must support that choice.

✦ The partner is there for support, not leverage. Therefore, it is essential to remember not to 'push' someone into poses that they would not typically go into on their own.

+ Communication is key. Ensure that you are willing to indicate to your partner when it is enough, when to ease off, or when to cease partnering.

+ Have a bell to use when it is time to stop and get students to listen to instructions.

+ It can help for partners to be around the same height.

+ Only add a few partner poses to your class unless it is advertised as a partner class.

+ Warm up physically with some flowing poses before partner work.

+ Consider doing the poses without a partner, e.g., traditional Camel and then with a partner, so students can observe the difference.

+ Demonstrate the poses with a partner first.

These poses can be used individually in your regular class or as a workshop. They are generally safer, beginner-level poses. Practise poses with a friend first before you teach them.

To Your Life

HEALING FROM STEALING

The opposite of steya is generosity. When we give freely without wanting something in return, we create an energy of abundance. What am I giving in this life? Where am I genuinely generous, and where do I hold back?

The opposite of steya is caretaking. When we look to our world and put into it what has been stripped out, we are giving back and creating a more equanimous relationship with Earth.

The opposite of steya is trust. When we trust there is enough to go around, we lose our tendency to take more than we need, and we fortify our sense of abundance.

It's natural to want what others have, to desire what we don't have.

Use these daily mantras as an antidote for steya.

I live a full and abundant life.
I have a generous, giving heart.
I trust there will be enough—that I am enough.
My heartfelt desire is for there to be enough for all living souls.
I am whole, and I need nothing else to complete who I am.

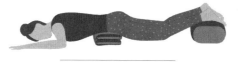

BRAHMACHARYA

BRAHMACHARYA

The same stream of life that runs through my veins night and day runs through the world and dances in rhythmic measures. It is the same life that shoots in joy through the dust of the earth in numberless blades of grass and breaks into tumultuous waves of leaves and flowers.

RABINDRANATH TAGORE

To the Mind

Brahma: god, energy, creative life force

Charya: to follow

This poetic-sounding yama means to walk as though god resides within you. When we live our lives feeling as though we are both divine and sacred, we are less likely to make choices that deplete our vital life force. If we practice brahmacharya, we become wise to squandering precious energy in the pursuit of unimportant or depleting actions. Like a squirrel storing nuts, we work at gathering our scattered prana, try to eliminate distractions, focus on what is essential, and practice yoga postures with consciousness to conserve energy while moderating or controlling what 'leaks' out of us.

To the Heart

Brahmacharya, the fourth yama, means to walk in tandem with the truth/god of your understanding. Historically, to do this, the student needed to conserve and preserve their life force so they could gather vitality to devote to their studies and practices. It was believed that through abstinence and celibacy, they could concentrate and contain their energy and therefore progress on the yogic path.

It is said that we all possess a secret life-preserving potion located at the base of the brain called *amrita*. This fluid of immortality is said to lengthen our life span. As it leaks out, it saps our energy. According to the ancients, merely turning upside down would preserve the fluid. Like a slowly leaking tyre, this yama asks us to look at the areas in our life where our 'amrita' or life force drains.

We practice yoga to fortify, preserve, and conserve our energy, not to deplete it. We also practice in order to plug the holes and the leaks, and to steer ourselves away from being exhausted or drained. Through self-examination, we may name the rivers of depletion that show up in our life. Excessive worry, needless running around, incessant talk, placing our energy into a goal that is not in alignment with our life path, and worshipping our addictions, are all stamina drains.

When we find a balance between energy coming in and life force going out, we are more able to pour our attention into the things that matter.

By eliminating distractions, not chasing after every pleasure, not getting caught up by the senses, and intentionally choosing where we concentrate energy, we are practising brahmacharya.

To the Body

❧ *Brahmacharya* ❧

Slow down and everything you are chasing will come around and catch you.

JOHN DE PAOLA

RESTORED AND CONTENT

Find sweet satisfaction and unparalleled comfort in this restorative sequence to preserve and reserve your energy.

SIX OPENING SEAL—SHANMUKHI MUDRA

To help block out the outside world, Shanmukhi seals off our sense openings—nose, eyes, ears, and mouth. It is a prelude to the practice of pratyahara, where we turn our focus inwards.

This mudra is performed with the fingers and thumbs:

- Place the thumbs in the ears.
- Place the index fingers over the eyes.
- Rest the middle fingers on the nostrils.
- Seal the ring fingers onto the lips.

Alternatively, to create a sense of comfort as if you were being swaddled, wrap a soft bandage around your forehead and eyes to 'seal' in your senses and deflect the outer world.

Can you hear the subtle internal sounds within you? Listen for the sound the yogis call *nada*, the sound of the universe. Additionally, practice Humming Bee's breath: Perform your seal and make a high-pitch humming sound in your throat.

HONOUR

1. Place a fold of blankets in the middle of your mat.
2. Place a bolster longways at the end of your mat.
3. Lie face down with your belly on the blankets and your feet on the bolster.
4. Place your arms in cactus shape.
5. Turn your head to one side.

EMBRYO

1. Place a bolster in the centre of your mat. Line up the short ends with the top and bottom of the mat.
2. Place a tightly rolled blanket or block underneath the top end of the bolster— your bolster should now be on an angle. You should be able to thread your arms under the bolster.
3. Kneel in front of the bolster.
4. Bring the bolster between your legs.
5. Fold your torso over the bolster.
6. Turn your head to one side.

PRONE TWIST

1. Keep the bolster set up the same as in Embryo.
2. Sit on the ground with your right hip to the bolster.
3. Bend both knees and stack your legs facing the left side of the mat.
4. Turn your body and place your hands on either side of the bolster.
5. Lay your torso over the bolster.
6. Turn your head and lie on your left cheek. If this is too strong, turn to face your knees.
7. Repeat on the other side.

SUPPORTED STRADDLE

1. Keep the bolster set up the same as Embryo or adjust its height.
2. Turn to face the bolster.
3. Take your legs apart and bring the bolster into your low belly.
4. Lay your torso over the bolster.

GODDESS

1. Keep the bolster set up the same as in Embryo.

2. Sit with your tailbone at the base of the bolster.

3. Bring the soles of your feet together.

4. Turn your knees out to the left and right; support beneath them with blankets if needed.

5. Lay your spine over the bolster.

SUPPORTED BACKBEND

1. Place the bolster in the middle of the mat. Line up the long side of the bolster with the top of the mat.

2. Place a rolled blanket at the top of the mat to support your neck and head.

3. Lay your mid-back over the bolster and place your neck and head on the support.

4. Let your arms fall out to the sides.

LEGS UP THE WALL

1. Set up the bolster as in Embryo.

2. Place one block on the tall height at the head of the bolster and one block on medium height to support the middle of the bolster.

3. Sit down with your right hip to the bolster.

4. Place a strap around your thighs tightly to hold your legs together.

5. At the same time swing your legs around to lie on the prop as you lay your torso onto your mat.

6. Your pelvis should be on the floor.

Brahmacharya

| 1 | SIX OPENING SEAL | 2 | HONOUR | 3 | EMBRYO | 4 | PRONE TWIST |

| 5 | SUPPORTED STRADDLE | 6 | GODDESS | 7 | SUPPORTED BACKBEND | 8 | LEGS UP THE WALL |

Teaching Notes

✦ Comfort is vital in all the postures. If the body is fully and adequately supported, it permits us to relax properly.

✦ Restorative yoga, as opposed to yin yoga, should have no or as little 'stress' on the joints or tissues as possible. We could consider restorative yoga the more yin version of yin itself.

✦ Restorative yoga is meant to 'restore.' The aim isn't to feel as much sensation as possible; the purpose is to heal and relax.

✦ When sequencing, consider the flow of the props and the movements to get from one to the other; the changeovers should be as neutral as possible.

✦ Be specific, meticulous, and careful with how you set your props up. Think of this as an intricate act of self-love. The props are the boundaries that you lean in to. They also create a container of comfort and care.

✦ This sequence uses minimum props, but extra blankets for wrapping, eye pillows, blocks, and bolsters will deepen the experience. The more ways you can prop the body, the more restorative the practice becomes.

✦ Like crawling under a blanket, the practice should be as quiet and dark as possible so the student can focus on their internal experiences.

✦ The body temperature will drop in restorative work, so provide warmth or blankets or extra clothing to accommodate this.

✦ Stay in the poses from four to fifteen minutes.

✦ Bring your attention to where you feel the most grounded, heavy, or connected to the earth; this is your anchor.

✦ Gentle movement can get the 'wriggles' out of students before settling into restorative yoga.

✦ Be reminded of the qualities of brahmacharya, of restoring and preserving energy.

✦ In flow or yang classes, concentrate on drishti to hone concentration. Reinforce the idea of mindfulness as an antidote to constant distraction. Remind students to come home when they find themselves staring at the mirror, giving themselves a pedicure, or darting their eyes around.

✦ Use forward folding postures to add to the theme of amrita leaking from the base of our skull; when we turn our heads down we retain this golden elixir.

To Your Life

+ Consider where you expend your energy daily. What are your go-tos? How much extra energy do you have when you abstain or omit unnecessary habits?

+ Consider how often you say yes when you already have a lot on your plate.

+ Setting daily intentions helps realign your vision and focus for the day.

+ Focus on what is important to you and what you value in life.

+ When you become unfocussed in a task, take a break so you can refuel and come back to it with fresh energy.

+ Are you able to find moderation in your emotions and your emotional responses?

+ Do you worry incessantly?

+ Energy flows where attention goes. Where do you put your attention? Is this how you want to spend your vital life force?

+ Look to where there is chaos or disorder in your life or home and consider ways you can organise these areas.

+ Some activities we use to relax, such as computers or TV, actually drain more energy from us. What is another way you can spend your relaxation time?

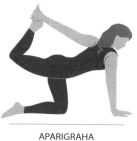

APARIGRAHA

APARIGRAHA

Peaceful is the one who is not concerned with having more or less.

RUMI

To the Mind

A: not

Parigraha: to grasp, grip, adhere, fixate, fasten, cling, or hold from all sides (anything) that is nearby

Aparigraha is the absence of greed, addictions, or grasping; appreciation and gratitude for what we have; and trusting in plenitude.

To the Heart

As humans, our natural tendency is to cling, store, or squirrel away what we have; from achievements to health, we are avid collectors.

We are the collectors of jobs, relationships, and possessions, which we store in the display cabinets of our psyche.

We are the accumulators of resentments and regrets, of unchallenged memories and unrealised ambitions, which we shove into the dark of our basements, hoping not to face.

We are masters of addiction to sugar, drugs, alcohol, technology, work, procrastination, self-doubts.

Letting go is having the courage to see the stuffed and stagnant versions of ourselves and choosing to exhale. It is the understanding that with conscious choice, we can allow what serves us to stay, and like the rain, let some of it wash away.

Letting go is one of the highest spiritual practices. When we remember that life is in constant flux and the world doesn't operate like a closed fist, we will loosen our grip on our storage systems and ultimately free ourselves.

To the Body

❧ *The Things That Bind Us* ☙

Let go or be dragged.

Zen Proverb

This practice works with binding. Binding is a metaphor for holding on. When we bind, tension and contraction are created; when we let go, there is a sweet release.

TENSE AND RELEASE SAVASANA

Contrast muscular tension or gripping with letting go. This dichotomy allows the practitioner to understand the duality of both states.

1. Lie down in Savasana.

2. Squeeze and release your fists. When you open them, feel the softness like a nest for a small bird.

3. Release and move your bottom jaw; feel the tendrils that hold it in place slacken.

4. Contract all your muscles—face, shoulders, hands, buttocks, legs, and toes.

5. Slowly release and let go with a sigh.

6. On your next exhale, release even more.

7. Repeat this whole-body squeeze and feel the flood of warmth as you let go of bodily constrictions.

KSEPANA MUDRA

Ksepana: to throw (away), to let go, to cast off.

Ksepana mudra is a hand gesture of letting go.

1. From Savasana, join your palms together and interlace all your fingers except the index fingers.
2. Cross your thumbs over one another.
3. Rest your mudra on your belly and point it towards your toes.

SUPINE HAND TO TOE POSE

1. Lie on your back.
2. Hug your right knee into your chest.
3. Lift your right foot to the sky.
4. Bind your right foot with a strap or take hold of the big toe with your second and third fingers. Alternatively, bind your hands like a hammock behind your thigh.
5. Relax your head and shoulders.

TIGER

1. Come to all fours.
2. Lift your right leg behind you. Keep your knee bent.
3. Press into your right hand.
4. Lift your left hand out and back to take hold of the right ankle.
5. Pull the foot in as you push the foot away to tighten the bow shape.

BOUND LUNGE

1. Step your right foot forwards into a lunge.
2. Interlace your hands behind you.
3. Press your palms towards one another.
4. Pull your arm bones back and down.
5. Open and spread your chest.

BOUND LIZARD

1. From Bound Lunge, release your bind.
2. Come down onto your forearms.
3. Turn your left forearm towards your right elbow.
4. Bend your left leg.
5. Take your right arm out to the right and around to clasp the left ankle.

BOUND FORWARD FOLD

1. Stand in Mountain pose.
2. Interlace your hands behind your back.
3. Come into a gentle Forward Fold, bending at the knees.
4. Let your arms and hands move towards the ceiling.

COW FACE EAGLE

1. Sit on the floor with your right knee stacked on top of the left and your shins folded back towards your outer hips.
2. Take your arms out to the sides, left and right.
3. Swing your right arm under your left, crossing at the elbows.
4. Turn your right hand so the palm presses into the left palm.
5. Repeat entire sequence on the other side.

The Things that Bind Us

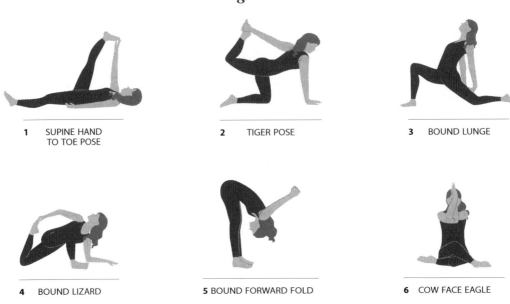

1   SUPINE HAND TO TOE POSE

2   TIGER POSE

3   BOUND LUNGE

4   BOUND LIZARD

5 BOUND FORWARD FOLD

6   COW FACE EAGLE

Teaching Notes

+ Incorporate progressive relaxation to shift holding patterns slowly. Use the tense and release technique (squeeze all the muscles in the body or parts of the body and slowly release the contraction).

+ Convey the idea to students that people think they are relaxed in the body and mind, but tension has made such a home, the new norm is holding on.

+ Mudras with interlaced fingers are symbolic of holding on. Our hands can release or clench. (See Ksepana mudra above.)

+ All yin practices hold the tenet of letting go deeply in each pose, and practice. When we hold muscular tension, we direct energy into the muscles as opposed to the connective tissue.

+ Binds of all forms demonstrate the tension that builds while we hold on and the sweet release when we let go.

+ When teaching binding sequences, remind students that achieving the bind is not as important as the feeling of the pose.

✦ Use straps and accessible binds, so students feel a sense of achievement.

Explore the range of binds

- standing
- seated
- balancing
- Warrior poses

Explore bind techniques

- bind hand to hand
- hand to body
- half binds
- full binds
- strapped binds

✦ Remind students that grasping, or parigraha, can be seen when we practice in the following ways:

- wanting the next pose
- wanting to look like someone else in your pose
- wanting to get to the next level of a pose too quickly
- injuring yourself by taking your body to an extreme end range of motion. The shoulder girdle is mobile but delicate and should be moved with mindfulness.

To Your Life

GRATITUDE PRACTICE

Gratitude practice highlights the sparks of happiness we experience day-to-day. When recognising the benevolence in others' actions, the preciousness and wonder of life, and the abundance of nature, we steer ourselves towards heartfelt generosity. Gratitude unties and blurs the borders between what we have and don't have, between grasping and giving away, and between holding on and the ability to let go.

When we are grateful for what we have, when we feel that there is enough to go around and we appreciate what is already in our life, we no longer have to grasp outside for the things that validate us.

Gratitude practices have been shown to activate the part of our brain that stimulates our reward and pleasure feelings.

Gratitude for Life

Thank you for this breath.

Thank you for this life.

Thank you for this love.

I acknowledge that life is a privilege.

I appreciate the immense beauty of this world.

I recognise that I have choices.

I honour my embodiment in all its shapes and forms.

On this day may I open to grace and all that life has to offer me.

THE ENERGY OF GRATITUDE

This series of appreciation starts from the foundations and moves to more subtle forms of gratitude. It could be used as a basis for a meditation or added to any practices involving the chakras.

1. I bring to mind the foundations from which I arose and am genuinely grateful for being given life in whatever form it was presented; it is a gift.

2. I am in awe of my body, how it allows me to give and receive, love and share, work and live my life, and without judgement of its shape or health I send it love and thanks.

3. I love and appreciate my strength, my courage and confidence to walk my path, to hold my head high, and my ability to stand up when needed.

4. I am grateful for the love I receive daily, the small acts of kindness, the generous, loving gifts of nature, creation, and all my relationships.

5. I send love and appreciation to all those who honour the world with healing, loving words and expressions. Thank you.

6. I appreciate and realise the importance of my insight, visions, and messages that I receive. May I be open to listening for them daily so that I can see with clarity and honesty.

∿∿ ∿∿ ∿∿
NIYAMAS

The niyamas are guidelines on how we tend to the body, mind, and spirit by refining the way we live. The practices shape our relationships towards ourselves and move inwards from the most tangible aspects of our being to an inner, deeper connection to our spirit.

If we tend to ourselves with love and care, form a lifelong commitment to practicing yoga, look at ourselves as if we were peering into a microscope, and have the grace to understand that we are not in control of every mystery in life, then we are working with the niyamas.

Just as in the case of the yamas, many different translations and definitions of the niyamas exist, including

+ the 'dos'

+ observances or duties we should direct towards ourselves

+ ways to respect ourselves

+ how we treat ourselves

+ self-conduct

There are five niyamas in Patanjali's *Yoga Sūtra*:

+ saucha

+ santosha

+ tapas

+ svadhyaya

+ ishvara pranidhana

The following section looks at these five principles in more detail and gives suggestions, practices and ideas about bringing the niyamas into modern day life.

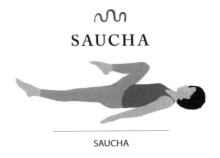

SAUCHA

SAUCHA

If with a pure mind a person speaks or acts,
happiness follows them like a never-departing shadow.

BUDDHA

To the Mind

Saucha: cleanliness or purity of the body, mind, heart, and soul. Saucha is the first niyama.

Saucha is the willingness to clean up our act. Metaphorically, we are decluttering the kitchen drawers, and sweeping our house clean. Cleanliness layers itself from the exterior to the interior, from the body temple to the soul temple. If we are to practice saucha, we must consider all parts of ourselves concerning this first niyama. The best place to start is with our senses or what we ingest through our eyes, ears, nose, skin, and mouth.

When we work towards cleanliness of the mind, body, and spirit, we gain lightness and vitality, and our energy flows more sweetly.

Kri: action or effort
Ya: soul

In Kundalini yoga, kriya, or set sequences of postures—breathing, eye gaze, and mantra—are used to obtain specific outcomes on the body/mind complex. Energetically daring us to move beyond what we think we can do, the kriyas help us burn through our blocks and limitations while at the same time moving latent energy up the spine and through the chakra system.

Like panning for alluvial gold, we continually have to sift the gravel from the pure metal. This distilling and processing is evident in Kundalini kriya work. The practices quite literally shake you up, move your energy, clear you out, and purify your being.

To the Heart

With saucha practices, we are trying to unveil our inherent essence, which is crystalline pure.

When a crayfish moults it blows itself up on the inside with water, forcing a split down the centre line of the old shell. It wiggles out of its old body, cleaning and disposing of the part of itself that it no longer needs. For a moment with its soft new shell, the crayfish is vulnerable, but this soon passes, and it becomes stronger than before.

Maybe we are moving through this life with a bursting shell that needs release, or its opposite, some stagnation that needs shaking up.

Every day we make choices about how to live our lives. These choices will either take us further away from our inherent purity or closer to it. Some of these choices are made on autopilot. If we are to live respectfully towards ourselves, it makes sense to choose conscious actions that lift our vibration and are in alignment with the value we place on our lives.

Once we start cleaning up our act, the things that are not needed or that clutter our lives will fall away. With clarity of body and eventually of mind, it becomes obvious which parts don't fit any longer. The whiter the snow of our life, the more obvious the stains become. The things that are in the way, our entanglements with the impure, will no longer grip us. We will then start to attract energy that will lift our frequency and bring us closer into alignment with what we desire.

To cleanse or clear the air between you and another person is the most difficult of cleansing practices. Anything left undone between you and another will veil your life. If you want to open your heart fully, you must not close anyone out.

Practising forgiveness and mercy cleans your heart and mind.

To the Body

᪥ *Saucha* ᪣

Try these energy shifting practices to lift and lighten your energetic field and thereby clean up your act.

SCISSOR LEGS

1. Lie on your back.
2. Place your thumbs under your sacrum and your hands flat on the floor to support your low back.
3. Lift both legs to the sky.
4. Lower your legs to a comfortable angle from the ground to prevent your back from arching.
5. Begin scissoring the legs.

LEG PUMPS

1. Lie on your back with your hands flat on the floor by your sides.
2. Bring your legs to Tabletop.
3. Start to pump your legs vigorously left and right like a hydraulic pump.

SEATED CAT-COW

1. Sit in Easy Seat pose with your legs crossed.
2. Hold on to your shins.
3. Begin Cat-Cow movements; keep a fast tempo.
4. Inhale, arch your heart forwards.
5. Exhale, round your back.

SEATED TWIST

1. Sit in Easy Seat pose.
2. ring your hands to your shoulders and lift your upper arms parallel with the ground.
3. Exhale, twist to the left.
4. Inhale as you twist to the right.
5. The breath is short and sharp, the movements staccato.
6. Repeat on the other side.

SIDE BENDS

1. Sit in Easy Seat pose.
2. Bring your hands to your shoulders with your fingers touching your neck.
3. Begin side-to-side movements, trying to move from the upper body.
4. Repeat for one minute.

PROPELLER ARMS

1. Clasp your hands in Bear Grip, with your fingertips interlaced and your hands facing each other.
2. Bring tension to your hands as you pull your fingers apart.
3. Inhale, lift your left elbow to shoulder height.
4. Exhale, lift your right elbow to shoulder height.
5. Continue this fast, vigorous pumping action with short sharp breaths for one minute.

SHOULDER SHRUGS

1. Sit in Easy Seat pose.
2. Inhale, lift your shoulders to your ears.
3. Exhale, drop your shoulders heavily.
4. Repeat this up-and-down movement for one minute.

NECK ROLLS

1. Imagine a flashlight on your skull.
2. Move your head in clockwise circles.
3. Move your head in anticlockwise circles.

Saucha

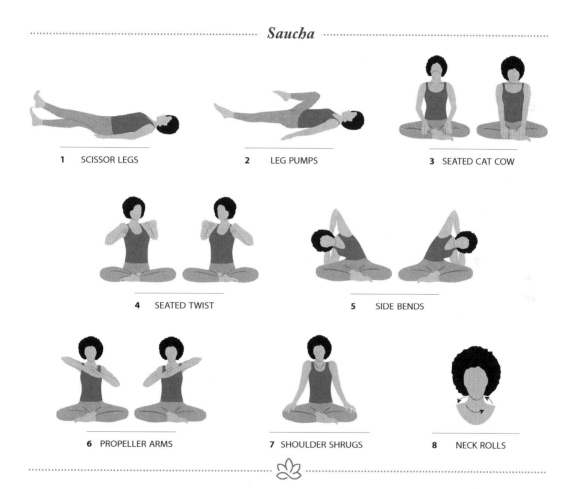

1   SCISSOR LEGS

2   LEG PUMPS

3   SEATED CAT COW

4   SEATED TWIST

5   SIDE BENDS

6   PROPELLER ARMS

7   SHOULDER SHRUGS

8   NECK ROLLS

Teaching Notes

+ The practices ask us to look at where we are resistant and move through that resistance. The place where we have the most resistance is often the place we need to work. As you practice, watch when resistance arises and see if you can move through that, even if only for ten more seconds.

+ Breath of Fire, or Kapalbhati, is one of the main breath techniques in Kundalini and can be done in many poses. Try Breath of Fire in Cat-Cow, Plank, and Down Dog, depending on your sequence.

+ If you are a vinyasa or power yoga teacher, try adding one or two of the exercises into the sequence.

+ Always make time to pause after the set to feel the energy shift.

+ In Kundalini it is believed we own a seed of latent power that sits at the base of the spine. The practices are designed to shift and lift this energy from the lower to the higher centres following the spinal chakra system.

+ The spine is considered the information highway in Kundalini. Consider designing your practice to move energy from the base to the crown. Start with lower grounding postures to activate and challenge the lower chakras, moving to the heart, then the throat and head.

+ Twists of all forms help to energetically and physically clean out our digestive system and the theme works well with cleanliness and saucha.

+ Sat Nam, meaning 'truth is my identity,' can be used in the practices to fortify the movement of stagnant energy. It can be chanted internally or externally.

+ See also Sufi Circles from air element practice.

+ Time the kriyas above for one minute.

To Your Life

Make friends with all parts of yourself, including your excretions that are vital for cleaning your body. Everything in us is there for a purpose. The practices below stem from the Ayurvedic tradition and centre around cleaning the eyes, mouth, and digestive system.

TONGUE SCRAPING

Scraping the tongue with a metal scraper in gentle downwards movements on waking removes the *ama*, or toxins, from the digestive system that build up overnight.

NETI POT

This small 'teapot' allows you to pour saline water into one nostril. The saltwater comes out the other nostril, cleansing your nose and sinuses.

LEMON WATER

A squeeze of lemon in warm water first thing in the morning energises and neutralises the digestive system.

TRATAKA

Light a candle and stare into the flame with soft eyes. The eyes will begin to water and self-clean.

CLEAN EATING

Eating food with high pranic value will not only lift your energy but also keep your body clean. Think of food as the information you are taking into your body. Ask yourself what value this food you are eating will have on the rest of your system.

High prana foods are fresh, minimally processed, and in season, and arrive to our plate soon after they were harvested.

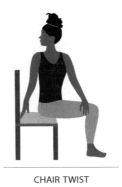

SANTOSHA

CHAIR TWIST

Seek contentment within yourself
Treasure the way your life is
When you understand your wholeness and your completeness
The universe belongs to you

LAO TZU

To the Mind

Sam/san: completely, wholly, entirely

Tosha: acceptance, satisfaction, contentment, sated, full, joyful

Santosha is the glass half full state of inner contentment. She is the comfortable feeling that arises when you make friends with all parts of yourself, while at the same time being at ease with what you don't have. Deeper and more permanent than happiness, santosha is a state of internal rest that warms you to your bones.

To the Heart

To be embodied is to experience itches that can't be scratched, abrasions that don't heal, and the nagging shadows of petty annoyances. Life niggles us in ways we don't care to mention or ways that we openly lash out against. It's an unstoppable roller coaster of highs and lows, the unknown, difficult yoga poses, and unsatisfying meals. It is a fault line of wrongdoings, and the sharp jabs of blame and shame.

But within the seed of shadows also lie bright lights. Without the suffering we wouldn't be able to experience the joy of this one wild ride.

There are satisfaction, treasures, and comforting dreams deeper than happiness itself. There are friendships and understandings and breakthroughs. There are apologies, comfort, and turnarounds. There are miracles and places of utter beauty.

Our choice is to run around spending precious energy trying to make our external world meet our internal desires—to get people to change, to change the world, to fix things, and acquire things to make us happy.

Or, we can use the power of mantra to pacify our cravings.

Can I be with this?
Can I accept this?
I am so grateful.
It is what it is.
Life is beautiful.
I am complete.
Everything is going to be okay.
This too.

We are stronger than we think. We have the capacity and power to shape our relationship to all of life's experiences. We can learn to love what is arising in all its complexity.

Santosha will naturally arise when you accept the challenge to live a full and human life.

When we fall in love with our lives, we understand the paradox, that where there is heartbreak there is love, where there is sadness there is joy, where there is hope there is despair. These are all parts of living in our human form.

So why not make friends with it all?

GOOD LUCK BAD LUCK

This parable illustrates the fruitlessness of control. Nature knows nothing of control; it simply marches to the beat of its own intelligent pulse. When we fall into the trap of what we think should be happening and try to steer our life in that way, we ignore the fact that life sometimes has other plans. We never know how the story is going to end.

We may not appreciate or like the present situation, but there may be a gift in it. Within acceptance of life lies santosha.

Once upon a time, an old farmer owned a single horse that one day ran away.
The villagers said to him, "Sorry for your news; this is such bad luck."
"Possibly," said the farmer.

The next day his one mare returned with three other wild horses.
The villagers said to him, "What wonderful news, you are so lucky."
The farmer replied, "Maybe."

His only son tried to break in the wild horses and was thrown off and broke his leg.
The villagers said to him, "What terrible news, very bad luck."
The farmer said, "Maybe."

The following week the military arrived to enrol all the able men for war, except for the son.
The villagers said, "I can't believe how lucky you are."
"Possibly," said the farmer.

To the Body

❧ *Santosha* ☙

Find support, ease, and contentment in this chair practice which can be adapted for the home, office, or studio.

EXTENDED MOUNTAIN

1. Sit comfortably on your chair.
2. Interlace your fingers.
3. Turn your palms away from your body.
4. Lift your palms to the sky and stretch through your torso.

CAT-COW

1. Place your hands on your thighs.
2. Inhale, press your chest forwards through your arms, arch your back.
3. Exhale, round your back, drop your chin.

SIDE BEND

1. Place your right hand on the chair seat next to your right thigh.
2. Lift your left hand into the sky.
3. Arch to the right.
4. Repeat on the other side.

TWIST

1. Place your right hand on the chair at the back of the seat or on the seat frame.
2. Turn to your right.
3. Place your left hand on your right knee.
4. Repeat on the other side.

SHOULDER OPENER

1. Sit forwards on the seat.
2. Grip the back of the chair where the frame meets the seat.
3. Turn the eye of your elbow forwards to rotate your arms outwards.
4. Press and lift your chest upwards.

FORWARD FOLD

1. Sit on the edge of the chair.
2. Take your legs about hip distance apart.
3. Lean forwards over your legs.
4. Let your body hang.
5. Place your hands on the floor or on blocks or behind the nape of your neck.

TWIST

1. Sit on the edge of the chair.
2. Take your legs about hip distance apart.
3. Place your right hand on the floor or on a block between your legs.
4. Open and twist your left arm and torso to the left.
5. Repeat on the other side.

SEATED PIGEON

1. Sit in the middle of the chair.
2. Place your right foot on the ground or on a block on the ground.
3. Place your left ankle on your left thigh.
4. Bend your left knee to 90 degrees.
5. Stay upright or lean forwards.
6. Repeat on the other side.

GODDESS POSE SIDE BEND

1. Sit in the middle of the chair.
2. Take your legs wide apart, turn out your feet.
3. Bring your right hand across your body and under your left thigh.
4. Hold the left side of the chair frame.
5. Reach your left arm into the sky.
6. Bow your body to the right.
7. Repeat on the other side.

CHAIR POSE

1. Sit on the edge or your chair.
2. Raise your arms up towards your ears.
3. Put your weight into your feet and lean your torso forwards a little.
4. Lift your seat off the chair.

HALF WAY LIFT

1. Stand up.
2. Turn and face the chair, stand about one of your foot's distance away.
3. Bend forwards and place your hands on the chair seat towards the back.

LEGS UP THE WALL

1. Lie down on your back with your sit bones near the edge of the chair.
2. Place your bent legs on the chair seat.
3. Place your arms by your side.

Santosha

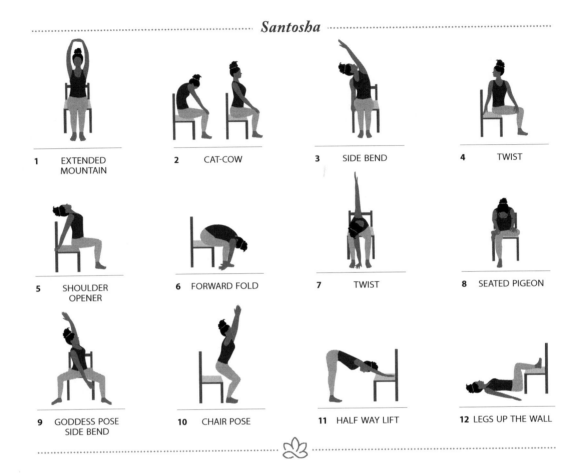

1 EXTENDED MOUNTAIN	**2** CAT-COW	**3** SIDE BEND	**4** TWIST
5 SHOULDER OPENER	**6** FORWARD FOLD	**7** TWIST	**8** SEATED PIGEON
9 GODDESS POSE SIDE BEND	**10** CHAIR POSE	**11** HALF WAY LIFT	**12** LEGS UP THE WALL

Teaching Notes

✦ The chair is a tool for all yoga practitioners. You can use the chair for support, for seated poses, for standing poses, or use it as a prop for restorative poses.

✦ Chair yoga is helpful for those with less mobility but also for those who sit a lot.

✦ Many poses can be adapted to the chair.

✦ The base of many poses in chair yoga is the sit bones and the pelvis, which is relatively fixed. Take care to avoid using the chair like a crowbar to twist deeply.

✦ All the dimensions you bring into your traditional classes, such as the arc of a class both energetic and physical, sequencing, and philosophy, also have a place in chair classes.

✦ Build strength and coordination by standing up and sitting down on the chair.

✦ When sequencing, consider the arc of any yoga class and adapt it to the chair.
- Centring: grounding, arriving, feeling into your body
- Setting an intention
- Arm movements coordinating with breath: Quarter Salutations
- Moving the spine in and out of its ranges of motion: twist, backbends, forward bends, lateral bends, and axial extension: Cat-Cow, Forward Fold, Twist, Side Bend
- Standing poses: Warrior One, Two and Three, Crescent Lunge, Triangle, Chair pose
- Balancing poses: Tree, Warrior Three, Half Moon
- Deeper twists, backbends, forward folds, or peak pose: Seated Head to Knee pose, Camel
- Cool down: Legs up the Wall, Pranayama, Meditation, Body Scan, Belly Breath,
- Seated Savasana

✦ Use blocks under your feet if your feet don't touch the floor.

✦ A yoga mat under the chair will keep the chair stable.

To Your Life

Discontentment can arise from two branches:
Getting what you don't want and not getting what you want.

Lesson five from Helen Schucman's book *A Course in Miracles* asks us to understand that the object, action, or person that has caused disharmony in us is not the real reason we are upset/dissatisfied/discontented. The lesson asks us to challenge our *samskaras* (habitual thought patterns through conditioning) with this sentence:

'I am never upset for the reason I think I am.'

It teaches us that whenever our peace is taken away, when we are worried, upset, angry, depressed, or jealous, to remember that the root of our distress is often not caused by where we point our finger.

As medicine, the course offers these practical mantras as a simple daily reminder that there is always more to being triggered than meets the eye. The practice is not intended to identify the cause of our dis-ease or to negate it, but to undo the braid of our samskaras so we can find more contentment and ease in our life.

I am not upset with _____ for the reason I think.

I am not angry with _____ for the reason I think.

I am not jealous of _____ for the reason I think.[13]

---

[13]Helen Schucman and William Thetford. *A Course in Miracles*. Foundation for Inner Peace, 2007. Reprinted with permission.

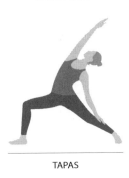

TAPAS

The man who moves a mountain begins by carrying away small stones.
CONFUCIUS

To the Mind

Tap: to burn through, flame, fire, friction, heat, fiery passion, incinerate, glow

Tapas is the inner resolve to bring about change in our life through consistent practice. Through self-discipline and willingness, we create 'heat' to burn through what is no longer serving us.

Tapasvin—austere practitioners of tapas

In India, *sadhus* or holy aspirants renounce their life and body in a type of spiritual detoxification. In an aim to rid themselves of their physical form they perform ascetic rituals known as tapas. Recognisable by their ashen painted faces, they will stand on one leg for twenty years until the muscles wither, or hold up one arm for their life, or vow never to lie down. They stand in the fire of the body by crossing the country on their hands and knees, prostrating and bowing in half salutations or fast intensely as a form of purification. In Hindu literature, tapas was considered intense preparation of the mind for ritual and supernatural acts.

To the Heart

Did you enter your life for comfort or for the complexity of evolution?

Change and evolution are messy, complicated, often painful, and require the friction of tapas, to go against the grain of how we usually act. This friction pushes us to our boundaries; it aches at our bones and rubs blisters into our palms.

To persevere, to show up for practice, to be disciplined, is tapas. When we willingly sit in the fire of self-transformation, we are turning our fear into fire and our excuses to ash. From here, there is no going back.

Take your seat.
Take a long slow breath in through your nose, right to the base of your belly. Stoke your fire to its core.
Block off your left nostril with your thumb or forefinger and breathe in fully through the right nostril to the midpoint of the brain.
Exhale slowly.
Continue to breathe in through the sun channel, as if you are piercing the sun with your breath.

Now bring to mind a consistent, non-serving thought that is standing in the way between you and creativity or love.
Write that thought on the paper of your mind. See it. Be deliberate. Now walk with it to the fire and throw it to the flames. See yourself marching steadily against the grain of old ways of being. Watch it burn.
Nothing can stop you now.

Rub your hands together vigorously. Feel the heat and friction.
Place your hands over your eyes, feel the warmth emanate.
When you are ready, slide your hands slowly to your lap and blink your eyes open.

To the Body

⤷ *Home Practice AM/PM* ⤶

Participating in daily practice is a way of moving from being a tourist of yoga into being a resident. Daily practice creates new neural pathways, breaks old habits, and enriches your yogic toolbox. Consistent practice provides a container for you to set your intention, or to start your day with understanding what is important to you. Practice will also prompt you to pay attention, reminding you to step away from the default of daily distractions. Cultivate tapas with these simple daily practices.

❧ *Home Practice* AM ☙

Morning practices benefit from

✦ intention setting.

✦ warming up the spine in all its planes of movement.

✦ salutations, to ward off sleepy energy.

✦ movement and strength-building poses.

✦ more vigorous breathing practices, especially ones that stimulate digestive fire.

✦ meditation, which may be substituted for Savasana.

························· *Home Practice AM* ·························

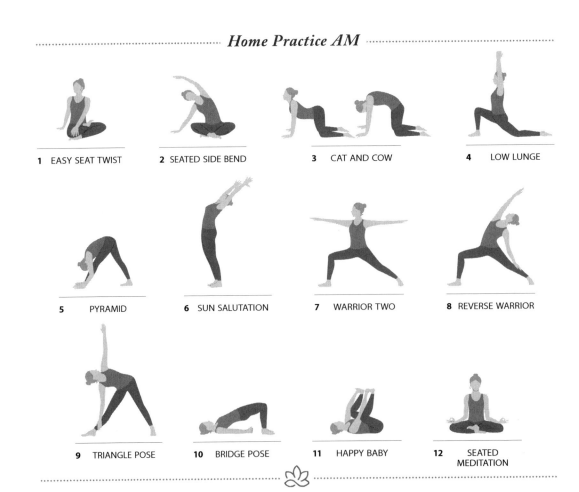

1 EASY SEAT TWIST   **2** SEATED SIDE BEND   **3** CAT AND COW   **4** LOW LUNGE

5 PYRAMID   **6** SUN SALUTATION   **7** WARRIOR TWO   **8** REVERSE WARRIOR

9 TRIANGLE POSE   **10** BRIDGE POSE   **11** HAPPY BABY   **12** SEATED MEDITATION

EASY SEAT TWIST

1. Sit comfortably with your legs crossed.
2. Inhale, lift up through your spinal column.
3. Exhale, twist to the right.
4. Place your left hand on your right knee.
5. Place your right hand on the floor behind you.
6. Repeat on the other side.

SEATED SIDE BEND

From Easy Seat

1. Place your right hand on the ground by your right hip.
2. Sweep your left hand over your head towards the right.
3. Repeat on the other side.

CAT AND COW

1. Come to Tabletop.
2. Inhale, drop your belly, lift your sit bones to the ceiling.
3. Exhale, arch your spine towards the ceiling.

LOW LUNGE

From Cat and Cow

1. Step your right leg forwards towards your right hand.
2. Lift your chest up and stack it over your pelvis.
3. Lift your arms to the sky.

PYRAMID

From Low Lunge on the right side

1. Frame your right foot with your hands on the floor or on blocks.

2. Lift your back leg up.
3. Move your front leg towards straight.
4. Bow over your front leg.
5. Repeat Low Lunge and Pyramid on the other side.

SUN SALUTATION

Move through a Sun Salutation of choice. See Salute the Elements for ideas.

WARRIOR TWO

From Down Dog

1. Step your right leg towards your right hand.
2. Turn your back foot flat.
3. Lift your torso and stack it evenly over your pelvis.
4. Lift your arms and hands to shoulder height.

REVERSE WARRIOR TWO

1. Slide your left hand down your left thigh.
2. Arch your right arm and torso towards the back of the mat.

TRIANGLE

From Warrior Two

1. Straighten your front leg.
2. Lean forwards and reach your right arm to the front of the room.
3. Tip your body.
4. Reach your right hand towards your shin, a block or the floor.
5. Repeat Sun Salutation to Triangle on the other side.

BRIDGE POSE

1. Lie down on your back.
2. Bend your knees and place your feet about hip distance apart.
3. Lift your pelvis towards the sky.
4. Interlace your hands under your pelvis, roll the upper arm bones out, and press into your upper arms.

HAPPY BABY

1. Bend your knees and hold the inside or outside of your feet.
2. Pull on your feet as you bend your knees towards the outside of your ribs.

SEATED MEDITATION

1. Come into Easy Seat pose.
2. Rest your hands on your thighs.
3. Be still, be at ease, and watch what arises on the movie screen of your mind.

❧ *Home Practice* PM ☙

Evening practices benefit from

✦ gratitude practices.

✦ cooling, calming breath practices.

✦ poses that negate a day of sitting.

✦ release of tension in the neck and shoulders.

✦ longer holds in hip-opening poses.

✦ yin style sequences.

✦ inversions.

✦ yoga nidra (yogic sleep) and meditation.

Home Practice PM

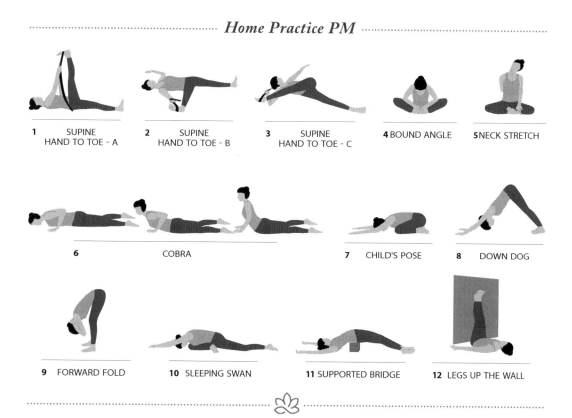

1   SUPINE HAND TO TOE - A

2   SUPINE HAND TO TOE - B

3   SUPINE HAND TO TOE - C

4 BOUND ANGLE

5 NECK STRETCH

6   COBRA

7   CHILD'S POSE

8   DOWN DOG

9   FORWARD FOLD

10   SLEEPING SWAN

11 SUPPORTED BRIDGE

12 LEGS UP THE WALL

SUPINE HAND TO TOE A, B AND C

1. Lie on your back.
2. Lift your left leg into the sky.
3. Loop a belt or strap over your left instep.
4. Hold the strap in both hands.
5. Soften your shoulders to the ground.
6. Stay here for five breaths.
7. Move the straps to your left hand.
8. Isometrically weight down your right hip.
9. Open your left leg out to the left.
10. Stay here for five breaths.
11. Lift your left leg back to the sky.
12. Swap the strap into your right hand.
13. Bring your left leg over to the right into a long leg Twist.
14. Stay here for five breaths.

BOUND ANGLE

1. Come to a seat and join the soles of your feet together.
2. Let your knees fall out to the left and right sides.
3. Hold your feet.
4. Bow over your legs.

NECK STRETCH

1. Come into Easy Seat pose.
2. Wrap your right hand behind your back and grasp your left arm.
3. Drop your head to the left.
4. Repeat on the other side.

COBRA

1. Lie on your belly.
2. Place your palms on the floor near your upper ribs with your elbows facing the sky.
3. Press into your feet.
4. Use the power of your core to lift your torso a little or a lot.
5. Lift and lower several times.

CHILD'S POSE TO DOWN DOG TO FORWARD FOLD

1. From prone, press into your hands, lift your seat, and press it to your heels.
2. Stay and breathe in Child for five breaths.
3. Press into your hands and lift your seat up and back to form an upside down 'V', or Down Dog.
4. Stay and breathe here for five breaths.
5. Walk your hands back to your feet.
6. Bend your knees and hold your elbows.
7. Bow over your legs.
8. Stay here and breath for five breaths.

SLEEPING SWAN

1. From Forward Fold walk your hands back out to Down Dog.
2. Lift your right leg into the air.
3. Bring your right knee towards your right wrist.
4. Lengthen your left leg out behind you.
5. Fold your torso over your right leg.
6. Repeat on the other side.

SUPPORTED BRIDGE

1. Lie on your back.
2. Place a block under your sacrum.
3. Stretch your legs out towards the front of the mat.
4. Stretch your arms over your head to the floor behind you.

LEGS UP THE WALL

1. Sit with your right hip close to the wall.
2. Lean back onto your forearms; at the same time swing your legs up to the wall and your torso to the mat.

Teaching Notes

+ Find a dedicated place you can practice.

+ Consistency is better than quantity. It is better to show up for two minutes each day than twenty minutes twice a week.

+ If you are not sure what to do, unroll your mat and sit on it. Be patient; something will arise. If you are still lost, consider taking your spine through its range of movements: forward folds, twists, backbends, and side bends.

+ If possible, a complete practice will include some mindful breathing and some meditation.

+ Vow to show up.

+ The moment you don't want to practice, and you do, this is tapas.

+ Tapas is not punishment. Discipline must be met with the principle of ahimsa or kindness.

+ Know what your roadblocks to practice are, and how they show up as excuses.

+ One of the biggest obstacles to daily practice can be an illness. Learn to adapt your practice to the changing conditions of your life.

To Your Life

You would think that as we evolve, once we understand and know ourselves better, then we would do better. But this isn't always the case. The concept of *prajnaparadha*, as offered by the Ayurveda tradition, is translated as 'offence against wisdom.' It means to go against the grain of what we know is authentic for us.

By ignoring our better judgement, wisdom, or innate guidance, we are led towards the path of suffering or ill-health. An everyday example is when we know we get tired or exhausted from staying up late, but we continue to do it anyway. Or we stay in a job that drains us, and we eat food that weakens us. We quite simply stop caring for ourselves even though we know deep down there are other ways.

Ayurveda and yoga teach that when you befriend your emotional, mental, and physical blind spots, you will ultimately know what is beneficial or harmful for you. You begin to draw circles around the lessons you are tired of learning, and from here, you naturally gravitate to the actions you should take to live a more peaceful life.

CHALLENGE YOUR HABITS

Habits that don't serve you are complacency wrapped up as safety. If we never challenge why we do something, then there is no need to change. The best way to check if you are acting from a mindless habit is to go without the action for a week. You'll quickly learn where you are attached.

+ If you always get up late, set the alarm and try getting up fifteen minutes earlier and do something valuable with that time.

+ Cultivate a daily practice of yoga, journaling, meditation, especially when you don't want to. Once you feel you have become disciplined, take this discipline into another field.

+ When you stick at something, this is tapas. Create endurance in your life by taking on a long-term or big project. To be successful, you need to finish it; separate success from failure with the willingness to keep trying.

+ Notice in your yoga practice where you want to give up, pit your mind against your body, and challenge yourself for the next breath.

+ The practices of mindfulness help us see where we are acting from snap impulse. Try delaying instant gratification by taking a breath in and out to linger a bit in the present moment before you act.

+ Watch your first movements for the day. By being attentive, we can see habit mind creep into our life. Do you reach for the phone as soon as you wake? Consider a new morning routine to claim your day.

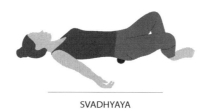

SVADHYAYA

SVADHYAYA

So you have to be your own teacher and your own disciple,
and there is no teacher outside, no saviour, no master; you yourself have to change,
and therefore you have to learn to observe, to know yourself.

JIDDU KRISHNAMURTI

To the Mind

Sva: self

Svadhyaya: self-study

Svadhyaya is learning about yourself to bring you to an understanding of your true nature. Through meditation, observation, enquiry, deep listening, and reflection we gain a richer sense of what it means to be human. Contemplating our life in relation to spiritual or inspirational texts will lead us deeper into the understanding of our many layers.

To the Heart

Deep within our psyche lies our unconscious blueprints laid down by our *whakapapa* (our ancestors and genealogical chain in the Māori tradition) and then by ourselves as we walk our path.

Svadhyaya is the practice of finding an alleyway into our intrinsic nature, to understand ourselves through observation, mindfulness, and study.

When we start to delve into the tide of our personal history and gain a snapshot of our patterns and conditioning, we will become less of a puppet to our loops of behaviour. It is from this that we can truly take ownership of how we live our lives. Non-judgemental study allows us to lean into our life and mindfully observe our actions, reactions, and tendencies.

When we take the time to sit and be, to examine ourselves and our life, we give ourselves permission and space to learn and grow.

Unconscious blueprints—samskara

In yoga, the term samskara has been likened to a hamster wheel that cements us in a loop of behavioural patterns. Like a tyre spinning in the mud, the more we spin, the deeper the rut becomes until we are stuck—the more we repeat a behaviour, thought, or action, the harder it is to break away. The only way out is to try something different. To step off the wheel, you first need to find a way to stop it turning.

The practice of yoga helps bring attention to your ruts and habits. When you lovingly lead awareness to your samskara, your relationship to it will change.

To the Body

❧ Self-Myofascial Release (SMFR) ☙

Myo: muscle

Fascia: responsive, intelligent connective tissue that runs in and around the muscles in a continuous network, giving us shape and form like an internal bodysuit.

Myofascial release is the general term given when we work the muscles and fascia to increase their health and hydration. Healthy connective tissue aids joint stability, helps us recover, and increases resilience within the body.

Release of tight or tender points in the body can be done through a variety of techniques including balls, rollers, massage, and pressure. When we apply pressure we stimulate the cells in the tissues to lay down more collagen and also increase their hydration, which leads to a healthier, more pliant fascia.

This practice uses balls, blankets, and blocks to release trigger points and fascial adhesions. Through self-study, the practitioner comes to know where they are tight or bound, what needs release, or where they are stuck.

If we take time to find our 'triggers,' we open the doorway to freedom from the knots of the body-mind.

SOLE OF FOOT

1. Stand up.

2. Place one ball under the sole of your foot.

3. Sweep the ball up and down the centre line.

4. Sweep the ball on the medial edge and the lateral edge of the foot.

5. Bring the ball to the centre of the foot and press down, either staying still or making small circles.

CALVES

1. Roll a blanket into a small cylinder; the tighter the roll, the more dynamic this becomes.

2. Sit on your calves with the roll between your seat and ankles.

3. After a minute, move the blanket to the fleshy part of the calf.

4. Move the roll to mid-calf.

5. Move the roll to behind the knee joint.

SACROILIAC JOINT

1. Lie in Constructive Rest with your knees together.

2. Place one ball on either side of the sacrum at the sacroiliac joints.

3. Stay here and let your weight fall onto the balls.

GLUTES

1. Move the balls farther out from the sacroiliac joint towards the side of your body about twenty centimetres.

2. Open your legs into Bound Angle pose.

3. Either stay here or gently open and close your legs.

GLUTE MEDIUS ROLL

1. Sit up and lean back on your arms.

2. Bend your left leg and straighten your right leg.

3. Place the ball under the middle of your right glute.

4. Use your arms to push you forwards and back over the ball.

OUTER HIP

1. Roll onto your right side and support yourself on your right forearm.

2. Bend your left leg and place your left foot on the floor to support you.

3. Place the ball on the outer fleshy part of the right hip.

4. Roll up and down. If you find a trigger point, stay on that spot.

TRAPEZIUS

1. Lie on your back.

2. Place a block under your sacrum, bend your knees, and place your feet on the floor.

3. Place two balls, one on either side of your upper spine at the base of your neck.

4. Cross your arms over your chest.

UPPER MID AND LOWER BACK

1. Remove the block but keep your legs bent with your pelvis and feet on the floor.

2. Move both of the balls down the spine a few centimetres. They should be on either side of your spine and inside your shoulder blades.

3. Do this three more times, exploring each station.

4. Try movements with your arms to intensify or change the sensation.

5. You will finish with the balls in line with the lower tips of your shoulder blades.

SUBOCCIPITAL RELEASE

1. Lie on your back with your knees bent.

2. Place a block under your head with the near edge on the bony ridge of your skull.

3. Roll your head to the right just by your ear. Either make a small left to right micro-movement or be still.

4. Move your head halfway between the right ear and the centre of the skull.

5. Keep moving your head, pausing and making micro movements until you reach the left side.

6. Make sweeping moves from left to right.

Myofascial Release

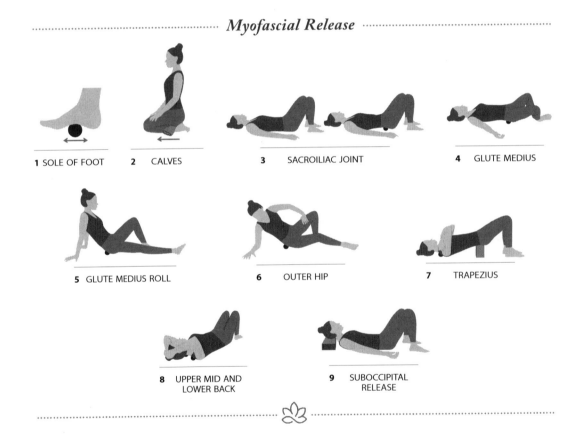

1 SOLE OF FOOT

2 CALVES

3 SACROILIAC JOINT

4 GLUTE MEDIUS

5 GLUTE MEDIUS ROLL

6 OUTER HIP

7 TRAPEZIUS

8 UPPER MID AND LOWER BACK

9 SUBOCCIPITAL RELEASE

Teaching Notes

+ The aim is not to beat your fascia into submission but to gently, over time, release held tension or trigger points along a line of fascia. Think little and often. Try not to pick on one spot in your body and massage that until you are sore or bruised.

+ Rather than gripping the prop with your body or mind, think release and acquiesce.

+ Intersperse movement, Savasana, or yin-style poses with the release. If you target one area, spend time releasing that area with a pose or movement. For example, if you do SMFR on the glute muscles, follow it up with Pigeon pose.

+ Think of the practice as bathing your nervous system. Keep your breath flowing and the approach soft. If it is too intense, you may be jolting your nervous system into the fight or flight mode. Try long, slow breaths while in the poses.

+ The prop shouldn't hurt or be on the bone or an injured area. Avoid painful areas.

+ If there is too much body weight on the prop try using another ball, block, or blanket to take some of the weight off the area you are working

+ There are many balls of different sizes, firmness, and feel; tennis balls work fine. Choose a size and firmness that feels beneficial.

+ The practice is not an exact science; it requires awareness, sensitivity, and investigation to find your 'spots' or trigger points.

+ If you have no equipment, the sections on Pada Bandha and Hasta Bandha have some SMFR ideas using your body as equipment. A rolled yoga mat can double up as a blanket.

+ Begin or end class with meditation so students can practice svadhyaya.

To Your Life

BE THE WITNESS—MEDITATION

The most potent way to see what we carry with us is through meditation. The act of sitting, noting, and letting go is a powerful way to glimpse our personal mysteries, inner dialogues, perceptions, and values.

Mindfulness meditation is the highlighter of judgements and self-doubts. But it will also let you see your dreams, visions, and deepest, most secret longings.

Sit comfortably.

Take a long breath in and exhale slowly.

Sit and witness what arises within.

Watch it all come and go without judgement.

Note, what is calling you today?

BE THE WITNESS—JOURNAL

The act of living gives us so many opportunities to study our impulses. How you do anything is how you do everything.

Today study the ways you meet your obstacles and challenges.

Where do you hold back?

When do you fight?

Where do you try too hard?

What triggers you?

Where do you give too much?

When do you give in?

When do you sidestep?

ISHVARA PRANIDHANA

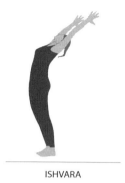

ISHVARA

God, grant me the serenity to accept the things I cannot change,
courage to change the things I can,
and wisdom to know the difference.

REINHOLD NIEBUHR

To the Mind

Ish: master, ruler

Vara: to choose

Ishvara: the spirit or higher power that you connect with, the divine intelligence that is your higher self, the guardians that tend to your life, god, buddha, a deity, nature, energy, that which you worship

Pranidhana: to give yourself over to, to dedicate yourself to

Japa mantra: a mantra consisting of a single word such as om, or a phrase such as om namah shivaya, which is repeated over and over again. The mantra can be recited internally or out loud and is often done with a string of mala beads. It is said that the repetition will break negative mental patterning and help focus the mind.

Kirtan: devotional chanting said to open your heart

Ishvara pranidhana, one of the three kriya yoga actions along with tapas and svadhyaya, is alignment with the divine. It is the connection to your higher self or god-like nature that lies within the heart of each one of us.

To the Heart

> *For we walk by faith, not by sight.*
>
> 2 CORINTHIANS 5:7

The last of the niyamas, ishvara pranidhana, asks for humility, faith, and a deeper understanding of our place in the cosmos. To stand outside on a starry night and gaze at the stars, or to press our feet into a million grains of sand, reminds us of a greater force that pervades nature and lies within us. When we align with our supreme divinity, we step into grace.

Pranidhana is the notion that we stop fighting the trajectory of our lives and leave some of the organisation to our guardians. It doesn't mean we don't try to make plans or that we are a puppet to fate, it means we have faith that things will be as they are intended to be, and someone or something else is tied into directing a beautiful life for us.

Sometimes, to live in ease, all we can do is choose to live with what is being presented.

Your innate wisdom will guide you if you listen; it will point the way on how to deal with your situations.

We don't have all the answers, we don't know how our life is going to project or play out, we can't see the future results of our present actions, so maybe the best thing we can do is to live our lives as best as we can with love and devotion to our work and relationships.

Have faith and surrender to the divine wisdom within you. Trust that it will know what to do and when to do it.

Slip out of control and into vulnerability.
Let down your walls and disarm yourself.
Find the place within where trust resides.
Sense its feeling tone.
Trust helps you onto the right path; where you stand now is where you are meant to be.
Trust hands you the relationships you need and takes them away when you don't.
Trust is the whisper of knowing what to do when you need to.
Cease the worry for your one sweet life.
You are adored and guided on your way.

ISHVARA PRANIDHANA IN ACTION

The love song to the lord, as the *Bhagavad Gita* is known, holds the divine essence of bhakti within its lines. This love and devotion that Arjuna has for Krishna is love in its purest form.

When Arjuna is broken into a million pieces because he doesn't want to kill his friends and family, he turns to the one he loves and asks, 'Please guide me.' Krishna urges Arjuna to practice ishvara when he says, 'Do your best, leave the rest up to me.'

Through devotional practices, service, chanting, and kirtan, bhakti practices aim to bond us closer to unconditional love in whatever form it takes. If we bathe ourselves in the sea of love, eventually the sea will disappear and there will only be love.

To the Body

Ishvara Pranidhana

This practice invites reverence, devotion, and connection to a higher energy. From chanting to mantra and graceful poses, it asks you to connect more deeply to the notion that we are divine beings living a mortal life.

CHANT OM

Om is the seed sound that holds us in the arms of greater love and wisdom. It is the primordial sound of the universe, and it represents all of creation. As you sing, let the sound arise from your heart or the place within you that represents ishvara. If you hold trouble in your heart, let this sound permeate your difficulty and for now, offer your situation into the vibration.

PUPPY DOG

1. Come onto your hands and knees.
2. Keep your hips over your knees and walk your hands forwards.
3. Rest your forehead or chin on the ground.
4. Bow your chest to the ground.

PRANAM MUDRA—COMPLETE SURRENDER

Pranam is a full-body prostration that connects us to the possibility of a higher power. It asks us to bow to the unknown and to give ourselves over to the practice, letting life force flow through us. Pranam inserted between or during Sun Salutations is a reminder of our interconnectedness with ishvara.

1. Lie on your belly and stretch your arms out in front of you.
2. Make Chin mudra by joining your thumb to your index finger. The index finger represents individual consciousness, and the thumb represents divinity. When we make this mudra, we tap into the innate wisdom of all consciousness.

CHILD'S POSE

1. From prone Pranam mudra, press your seat back to your heels.

2. Stretch your arms out and bow your head to the floor.

3. After ten breaths, lift your torso so your shoulders are over your hips. Sit on your calves and prepare for pranayama.

BREATHE—SOHAM

So: that. 'That' means the universe, creation, or the source of your spiritual inspiration

ham or hum: I am

Soham or sohum meditation is a powerful yet straightforward mantra to concentrate the mind using the breath. The mantra is said to bring you into direct connection with all of creation. Using this meditation allows us to feel connection and interconnection to the source of all things and all that walk this earth.

As you breathe in, silently focus on the word 'so.'

As you exhale, feel the word 'hum' internally.

Feel as you repeat the words that you are merging with the divine, consciousness, or a higher power. If you prefer, you can imagine that you are connecting with all of humanity.

Let the words wash through you and over you.

COSMIC MUDRA

This mudra is often used in Zen practices, to connect us to the cosmos.

1. Sit comfortably and turn both of your palms up. Place the left hand on top of your right open palm.

1. Join your thumbs to form a ring.

2. Relax your shoulders.

Close your eyes.

Take your attention inwards.

When you join your thumbs, you are tapping into the universal soul, the cosmos, and all of creation.

As you press your thumb tips together, feel yourself start to surrender to the pull of a higher, guiding force in your life.

Relax. Let go. Trust.

Is there is a situation in your life now that you feel you need to fix, control, or alter? Can you make peace with it and allow it to unfold?

We can't always see the finishing lines, but we can learn to be at peace with not knowing.

FAITHFUL SALUTATIONS

Invite students to do quarter, half, and full salutations with their eyes shut. Trust they will know what to do. See 'Air Salutations' for instructions.

Inhale, and God approaches you. Hold the inhalation, and God remains with you.
Exhale, and you approach God. Hold the exhalation, and surrender to God.

T.K.V. DESIKACHAR

LOW LUNGE BACKBEND

1. Exhale, step your left leg to your left hand and drop your right knee to the floor.

2. Inhale, lift your chest, shoulders, and arms so they are stacked over your hips.

3. Exhale, take your hands behind your back and interlace your fingers.

4. Inhale, lift your side waist and sternum.

5. Exhale, bow back.

LOW LUNGE SIDE BEND

1. Undo your hands.

2. Lift your right hand to the sky.

3. Exhale, arch your right hand over to the left. Let your left hand drop farther to the floor.

4. Inhale, bring your chest back to neutral and both of your arms to the sky.

LOW LUNGE TWIST

1. Exhale, plant both hands on the ground on either side of your left foot.

2. Inhale, open your left arm to a twist.

LOW LUNGE MONKEY TAIL

1. Exhale, point your left hand and arm to the back of your mat.

2. Inhale, bend your right knee and bind your hand to your right foot.

3. Exhale, stabilise into your right hand and shoulder joint.

4. Inhale, twist your heart up to the sky.

HALF MOON TO SUGAR CANE

1. Place a block on the floor forwards of and outside your right foot.

2. Place your right hand on the block.

3. Lift your left leg into the air.

4. Stack your left leg and hip over your right leg and hip.

5. Stay here for two to three breaths.

6. Bend your left knee, so the heel touches the left glute.

7. Bind your left foot with your left hand.

8. Arch and press your chest forwards.

9. Repeat entire sequence from Sun Salutation on the other side.

Ishvara Pranidhana

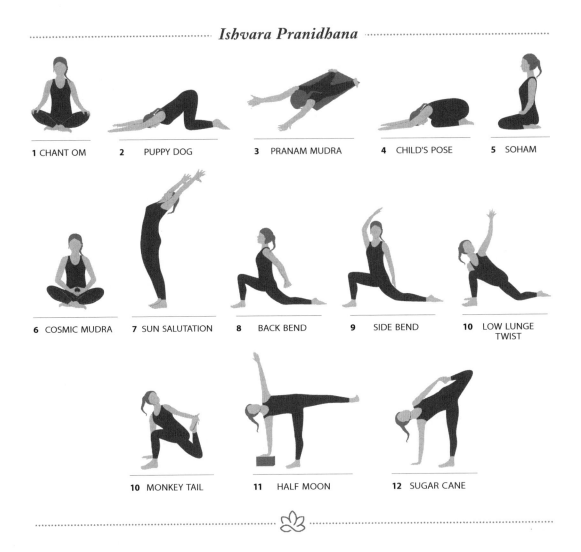

1 CHANT OM **2** PUPPY DOG **3** PRANAM MUDRA **4** CHILD'S POSE **5** SOHAM

6 COSMIC MUDRA **7** SUN SALUTATION **8** BACK BEND **9** SIDE BEND **10** LOW LUNGE TWIST

10 MONKEY TAIL **11** HALF MOON **12** SUGAR CANE

Teaching Notes

✦ Consider approaching salutations with the idea of your body as a moving prayer or offering. With each breath, surrender to whatever you equate with your higher self, your guardian, or ishvara.

✦ Closing your eyes during simple opening moves or a salutation gives you a different perspective on your practice, moving you from what you do to what you sense and feel. It helps us remember our unique navigational system that is keeping us safe.

+ Inserting full Pranam after Chaturanga gives the student a chance to remember the concept of devotion.

+ Anjali mudra is the recognition that we are connected as a human family through love. It means, 'I honour your divinity, I bow to you.' Use Anjali mudra in your poses to remind students of their connection to the spark of divinity within us all.

+ When you move into postures, expand outwards from the heart centre. Make the physical heart, chest, and arms a physical magnet for divine love and inspiration.

+ Any poses that mimic bowing, such as Forward Fold, standing Wide Leg Straddle with your head on a block, Child's pose, or Easy Seat fold, remind us that when we bow we perform a body metaphor of pranidhana.

+ Japa mantra or kirtan will instil the devotional element of bhakti and ishvara.

+ God is whatever form of love or spiritual inspiration we decide. It could be a pet, a loved one, a deity, your garden, wherever you feel peace and radiant love in your life.

To Your Life

Anything that you devote yourself to and that connects you to the higher part of yourself evokes ishvara pranidhana.

+ Practice karma yoga—the act of being of service to others without expecting return for your work. This practice is closely intertwined with the practices of bhakti.

+ Create an altar towards the deity that calls your heart the most. Consider what you want to put upon this sacred space. Find something to represent gratitude, compassion, inspiration, love, and devotion.

+ Rub your hands together vigorously to generate energy and life then place the hands over your eyes. This symbolic gesture will help remind you to let go of control because your eyes are covered, and to trust more fully.

+ Movement, dancing, and creativity are ways to feel the power of ishvara move through you.

+ Study stories of the gods and goddesses, or study the life of an enlightened spiritual being.

+ All forms of meditation are an act of devotion.

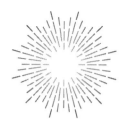

CHAPTER SEVEN

DIVINE ENDINGS

The way we end our class is what will live on in the hearts and minds of the student. When everything has fallen away, when we have been stripped bare and made whole, we get a glimpse of who we are. As Carl Jung says, to become who you truly are is the privilege of a lifetime.

That moment when you hear the sweet word 'Savasana' and you willingly lay yourself down to be held by the earth, you know you have arrived. In many ways Savasana is the peak pose of any class, a seemingly simple shape, but hidden in the shape we meet the difficulty and complexity of stillness.

Savasana is not just a pose; it is a state. It's important to be led by the hand slowly down the hallways of the body, breath, and eventually mind, so we can become one with the pose.

Relaxation is a conscious choice to listen to ourselves, as opposed to distracting ourselves. Distraction takes us further away from peace; conscious relaxation opens the doors to peace.

This relinquishing of the body/mind is the symbolic bodily gesture of death to our egos, our desires, and our grasping. When we lay the body down in this way, we pay respect to the practice, and we pay respect to ourselves as it slowly but surely downloads into our being.

This section pays tribute to the stillness of Savasana and its importance in our worlds of busyness and pursuit.

Here we get to wipe the slate clean and end our yogic odyssey.

Before we begin again.

STILLNESS IN MOTION—SAVASANA

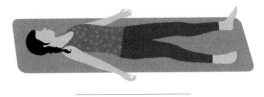

SAVASANA

*Now we will count to twelve
and we will all keep still.*

*For once on the face of the earth
let's not speak in any language,
let's stop for one second.*

PABLO NERUDA

Sava: corpse

Mrtasana: Corpse pose

Savasana can be used

✦ as a guide to induce tamasic or relaxed energy.

✦ as a precursor to yoga nidra.

✦ to ease the body and mind of sleep debt.

✦ to help enter the delta (dreamless) state.

✦ to begin and end a class.

All of humanity's problems stem from man's inability to sit quietly in a room alone.

BLAISE PASCAL

Krama: steps or sequence

THE KRAMA OF SAVASANA

1. Physiological relaxation

Spend the first five to seven minutes getting ready for the state of Savasana. We lie down, move a little, get settled, then we are prepared to receive. Use progressive relaxation techniques, such as squeezing and releasing the muscles. (See also Movements into Savasana.)

2. Pratyahara

During this state, we start to draw our senses inwards and are no longer distracted by the outside world. It is a feeling of non-obligation where we drop all our to-do lists or the need to be somewhere else. A sense where you no longer want to leave Savasana may start to surface, as if you were glued to the floor and can't get up. You also may hear the voice of the teacher drift in and out of your awareness, but you no longer want to react to any external stimuli.

3. Shunya

Shunya means emptiness; ashunya means not empty. You only know you have achieved this state of emptiness after the fact. You have a feeling of having "returned" from somewhere. Your teacher might have had to 'wake' you, but you know you weren't asleep.

The hardest work of all is to do nothing.

PROVERB

KRAMA ONE—THE BODY RELAXES, THE BREATH SOFTENS

Bring awareness to the softness of your skin,
the texture of your clothes,
your jigsaw bones—their lengths and turns, the spaces in between.
Feel gravity's heaviness in the back body,
lightness and freedom on your front.
Where is there symmetry, where is there an imbalance?
What is holding you together, is it tension or ease?
Now your breath.
Is it slow or fast, is there movement in your ribs or belly?
Notice your coexistence with your life force.

KRAMA TWO—PRATYAHARA

In this stage, withdrawal from the physical world will start to occur, but we are still aware of our surroundings. Our interaction with external stimuli lessens, and we become nonreactive to sounds and stimuli as they occur. We lose curiosity and ambition.

Here, energy is directed into the parts of the body that need it the most for healing and repair and growth.

Feel your body lying in the room.

Without opening your eyes, sense the four walls, the ceiling, and the floor.

Imagine your body lying on the floor as if you were looking at it from above.

Take your attention to the sounds outside of you.

The sounds far away.

And those close to you.

Now imagine you have floated above your body and you are looking at yourself lying on the floor.

See the energy that surrounds you.

Lie here and be aware of yourself lying in love with the world.

KRAMA THREE—SHUNYA

In shunya you will feel an emptiness or void, as if you have left your body. It is the free dive into the deepest part of the ocean, and it is here the saline drop of your body dissolves into the silent sea.

Savasana

⊙⊙

THE POSE OF SAVASANA

In stillness all the secrets of eternity will be revealed.

LAO TZU

Getting people into Savasana is an art and a science. You want the student to be comfortable, so they don't fidget, and so it is important to support any injuries or tightness. The entry into Savasana should feel safe and warm for the student. When we feel at ease and protected, we are more easily able to practice the skills of quietness, stillness, and introspection.

✦ The chin and the forehead should be about in line. When the chin juts upwards, the mind won't rest as well.

Lie down on your back and adjust your head so the forehead and chin are parallel to the ceiling to create room in your throat. You may need a thin blanket under your head.

✦ The shoulder blades should lie flat on the back.

With your knees bent, push your feet forwards a little to move your shoulder blades down your back.

✦ The chest should be open and broad to allow spaciousness and softness for the lungs.

Widen the sternum like it is being pulled apart and lengthen the low ribs towards your feet, as if you were drawing a shutter closed.

✦ The back of the body should feel weighty and broad.

Feel the west or back side of your body spread to the edges of your mat.

✦ The spine should maintain its natural curves.

Ensure your spine still maintains its four curves on the floor. Feel free to place a rolled blanket under your knees if the low back flattens.

✦ The arms should be relaxed on the floor with the palms turned up.

If the palms turned up feels constricting in the shoulders, place your hands on your belly or turn the palms downwards. Support your shoulders with a blanket if that brings more ease.

✦ The legs should lengthen out from the pelvis.

Press forwards through your heels to lengthen the backs of your legs and then let your feet turn out (or in) and become heavy like two stones.

MOVEMENTS INTO SAVASANA

The times are urgent—let us slow down.

BAYO AKOMOLAFE

Starting your class in Savasana allows students to release the day physically and mentally. The posture supports the back, fully helping to align the spine. Finishing in Savasana bookends the class and raises spirits before we enter back into our life.

This series of movements help relax and settle the body before Savasana, removing any 'gremlins' from the day.

HEEL ROCKS

1. Lie down.
2. Point and flex your toes on both feet.
3. Start slowly then gain momentum then slow down again until the movements are almost imperceptible.

LEG AND LOWER BACK STRETCH

1. Lie down.
2. Press through your right heel.
3. Stretch your right leg as far away from your pelvis as possible.
4. Feel the move come from your low back.
5. Return your right leg to neutral.
6. Stretch your left heel forwards.
7. Go back and forth until you feel your lower back release.

PELVIC HALVES

1. Lie down.
2. Bring your right knee to 90 degrees along the floor like a 'cactus' leg.
3. Move your right arm to 90 degrees like a 'cactus' arm.
4. Arch through your left side.
5. Slide your right arm back to shoulder height and your leg back to its original position. The arm or the leg doesn't come off the floor.
6. Repeat on the other side.

CROSS LATERAL STRETCH

1. Lie on your back like a starfish or snow angel with your hands and arms outstretched.
2. Take a breath in and stretch your right foot forwards on the floor on a diagonal while extending your left arm back on the floor on a diagonal.
3. Repeat on the other side.

TENSE AND RELEASE

1. Lie down.

2. Squeeze your hands and fists tightly, hold, now slowly release.

3. Squeeze the muscles of your arms and legs, hold them tight; as you release them feel the warmth.

4. Squeeze your whole body tightly, hold, hold, hold, now release slowly.

BREATH RELEASE

1. Inhale through your nose.

2. Open your mouth and let out a long slow *HAAAA*.

Movements into Savasana

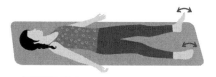

1   HEEL ROCKS

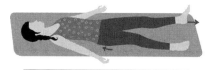

2   LEG AND LOWER BACK STRETCH

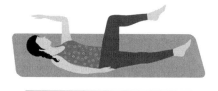

3   PELVIC HALVES

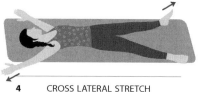

4   CROSS LATERAL STRETCH

SAVASANA POSITIONS

PILLOW

If you have a bolster, place this under the secret crook at the back of your knees. Bending your knees takes weight out of the legs and the tension from the back of the legs. Softening at the knees allows the pelvis to drop more heavily and the breath to free up.

Place an eye pillow over the eyes.

THIGH STRAP

Place a looped strap around your thighs. Put some tension into the loop and lie down with your legs outstretched. The belt will keep your legs close together but support them at the same time.

WEIGHTED DOWN

Have someone weight you down with blankets and sandbags.

Place a blanket over the upper half of the body and firm it down around the shoulders as if you were tucking a loved one into bed.

Place an eye pillow over the eyes.

Weight the legs, arms and hands.

BABY SAVASANA

Lie on your side with a folded blanket under your torso.

Place your head on a pillow.

Fold the top leg to right angles and place it on a bolster.

Sava-Asana

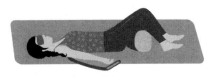

5   PILLOW

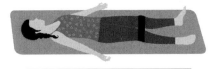

6   TIGHT STRAP

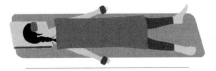

7   WEIGHTED DOWN

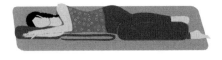

8   BABY SAVASANA

ෆ෬

SAVASANA ENHANCEMENTS

If it's appropriate for your student, you may wish to try these body-melting adjustments. Remember to leave some time and space in Savasana for the student to be at peace.

EYE BANDAGE OR FOREHEAD MASSAGE

Massaging the point between and slightly above the eyebrows softens the lines of tension here. This indicates to the brain that all is well, and it can quieten and relax. A soft gauze bandage wrapped around the eyes and head or an eye pillow will produce a similar effect.

LEG ROCK

Bend your knees and pick up the student's legs; they need to relax fully so you can feel the entire weight of their lower half. Gently swing the legs to the left and right like a pendulum. Slow down the pace and make it more subtle as you lower the legs to the floor. Place your palms on their inner feet and apply a little pressure to seal their feet down and help release their legs in an outwards direction.

SHOULDER SNUGGLE

Pick up the right arm with your left hand. Shake the arm a little to encourage the student to let go. Bend your knees and use your right hand to reach under the shoulder blade. With a scooping action lift the shoulder blade, pull it slightly towards their right waist and set the arm and hand down away from the body. Repeat on the left side.

OCCIPUT MASSAGE

Pick up the back of the student's head and cradle their neck. Pull your fingertips back until you feel the bony ridge of the occiput. Massage this area with your fingers before placing the head down to rest.

TEMPLE AND BROW MASSAGE

Cup your hands over the student's ears. Move to the temples with your middle fingers and softly massage. Use your thumbs to stroke the hair on the eyebrows away from the centre line. Finish by bringing your hands into namaste and touching your little finger lightly on their third eye.

WORDS TO GUIDE

ARRIVING

Lie in balance

Tend to yourself

Yield into your body

Sense gravity and levity

Feel heaviness and release

Have a willingness to let go

Allow yourself to be held here

Explore any sensations arising

Savasana is relaxation in action

Connect to the quietest part within

Relinquish the need to do anything

Peace rushes in as you become still

Lay yourself down on a carpet of petals

Let the pull of gravity settle you earthbound

Lay your body down like a fallen parachute

EYES, EARS, HEAD, BRAIN

Deepen your temples

Let your brain fall back and down

Liquify the point between the eyes

Let your inner ears soften and deepen

Soften the point between the eyebrows

Take your attention to the point between the eyebrows

Let the bony landmarks of your face, cheeks, eye sockets smooth

MOUTH, JAW, TEETH, TONGUE

Feel the teeth float in the gums
Melt the base of the jaw
Feel the tongue widen and spread in the mouth
Release the tongue from the root of the mouth
Soften your upper palate

HANDS, FEET

Feel your fingers furl as if you were holding a small bird
Weight your toes like ten small pebbles
Let your feet turn of their own accord

RELEASING TENSION

Ease yourself into Savasana
Release the holding patterns
Dissolve tension in the body
Drop the holding patterns of tension within
Feel your liquid-like honey insides soften and melt

WHOLE BODY, SKELETON

Drape your body like fine silk cloth
Relax the soft marrow of the bones
Let the front of the body be light and receptive
The back of the body is heavy and broad
From the centre of your body spread out
Move inwards from the surface to the contents
Feel where your skin is soft and where it is stretched

ENDING WORDS

Linger here for as long as you wish
Lie here and enjoy what you have created
Nourish yourself in this sweet posture until you feel a need to rise

SAVASANA POETRY

ON THE MAT
Practice poses to work with your history
Practice breathing to work with where you are now
Practice meditation to guide your future
Practice Savasana to let it all go.

NOTHING
Nothing to do
Nowhere to go
Nothing is broken
No one needs fixing
Nothing needs changing
Everything is perfect

EARTH SUPPORT
Lie down on the floor and spread your body as if you are lying on a carpet of newly fallen soft spring petals.
Feel as if you are being held in the great Mother's arms with her gentle support beneath your head, spine, and legs.
Just as the ground holds your weight, are you willing to relinquish the weight of your world into the ground?

Hover your left foot off the floor.
Feel the weight and heaviness of your left foot and leg.
Drop the foot to the floor.
Feel the sweet release.

Lift your right foot off the floor.
Feel the weight and heaviness of your right foot and leg.
Drop the foot to the floor.
Feel gravity and release with each lifting and relinquishing.

Hover your right hand and arm.
Feel the weight of your hand and arm. Put all your attention into the weight.
Drop your limb to the floor. Feel the release.

Lift your left hand and arm.
Feel the weight of your left hand and arm. Put all your attention into your hand and arm.
Drop your limb to the floor. Feel the release of weight.

Feel your arm bones turn in their sockets and spread like angels' wings as your collar bones internally widen and fall like branches into the soil.

Lift your head.
Feel its heaviness. Put all your attention into the weight.
Place your head to the floor gently.
Feel the release.

Your whole body, weighted, warm, held, and supported by the earth.
Finally, rest all parts of yourself to the earth.

SURRENDER TO GRAVITY

Lie down.
Surrender yourself to gravity.
Close down the blinds of your eyes.
Feel the intimate harmony and connection of your precious body to the floor.
Each point of contact is a chance to feel more supported,
And each breath a chance for the earth to move more deeply into your being.

REPLENISH

Lie down with as much love as you can.
Feel the earth receive you.
Lie there like a fallow field, resting, at ease.
Take a long slow inhale and imagine that you are being replenished.
As you exhale, give this breath back out into the world.
Savasana.

HONEY

Melt and spread yourself onto your mat.

Imagine your body is filled with viscous honey sinking into the pool of gravity.

Let this golden mess spread across the floor as the back of the body grows broader.

Above you is a warm, soft glow that coats your skin as if someone has placed your favourite blanket on you.

Each breath, slow, soft and sweet, taking you deeper and deeper into yourself.

LET GO

Let your bones settle into the heartbeat of the earth.

Let go of all sending and settle into storing.

Let go of all borrowing and settle into returning.

Let go of all transmitting and settle into absorption.

SINGING BOWL

Let your mind rest where your head falls.

Close down your eyes and turn inwards to the dark stillness within.

Hear the sounds around you start to drop away into the background, just as the bird's song fades at the turn of the day.

Listen to the singing bowl. (Strike the bowl)

Hear the strike, the resonance, and the fade.

Follow the sound right to its limits until you hear silence.

INK

Lie in Savasana with your arms by your sides, so your shoulders feel comfortable.

Press a little into the back of your head so you can snuggle your shoulder blades down like flat river stones on the earth.

Open your hands and turn your palms up. Your fingers furl slightly as if you were holding a lost bird.

Let your body spread and widen in ever-increasing circles as if you had dropped ink onto blotting paper.

Feel the bones give up their work of holding you upright as gravity spreads you deeper and deeper into the earth.

SUSPENDED

Lay your bones onto your mat.

Take a long slow breath into your body matrix; as you exhale, feel a warmth of relaxation flood you.

Take your attention to your skin. Feel how it coats your entire body, holding the bones in place.

Now dive down under the skin and feel into your skeleton, all the bones that make up your shape. The skull, the arms, the rib cage, the hips and legs.

As I name the bones, imagine each one is floating and suspended in water, being held on the tide of soft tissues.

Skull, jaw, collarbones, upper arms, lower arms, all ten fingers.

Sternum, rib cage, front of the pelvis, back of the pelvis.

Upper thighs, lower thighs, all ten toes.

Your entire skeleton is floating, supported and suspended.

Savasana.

THANK YOU

Pour your attention into your still body.

Gather your awareness behind your breath.

Turn up the volume of receptivity, openness, and acceptance.

Feel a deep sense of release, wholeness, and peace.

Be present to yourself, for yourself, just as you are.

Thank yourself for showing up today.

CLOSE YOUR EYES

'Close your eyes.

Fall in love.

Stay there.'

—Rumi

ROLL UP YOUR MAT

I close my eyes to old ends. And open my heart to new beginnings.

NICK FREDERICKSON

In that last minute, as Savasana comes to an end, everything is perfect. For a moment, there are no arguments, no heartbreaks or loss, no messiness to life. You will see this evidence collected in the Sava bodies. These delicate seconds are the perfect time to remind our class of what they know already. It is here we set sail our final words into their communal hearts and spirits and midwife the yogis into their day.

These words can be uttered

+ at the end of Savasana, when students are still lying down.

+ when students have rolled over to their sides before coming to a seat.

+ when students have returned to a seated position, just before the class ends.

Teaching Notes

+ Consider what you would like to do prior to Savasana, post-Savasana, or as a substitute for Savasana. A yoga class could be ended in a restorative pose, with meditation, or with pranayama. What time of the day and how much time you have will dictate what you can fit in. Pranayama ideally fits before meditation. *Posture-breathing-sensory withdrawal-concentration-meditation* is the prescription from Patanjali.

+ Try not to rush your ending. Leave plenty of time for Savasana and at least a minute to get up out of Savasana to a seat.

+ Decide on a closing ritual. How you can layer your last few words of your theme while taking students into and out of Savasana will make a lasting impact on your teaching. A good ending will strengthen all parts of the class, even the parts you felt didn't land well.

+ How do you want students to remember the class? What words or flourish do you want to drop into the final moments? The ending is crucial. It is what students will leave with, and if it is sweet, or bittersweet, it will stay with them for a lot longer. If you are not sure what to say try finishing this sentence, 'May this practice (plus a reference to your theme)'.

✦ At the official end, sit silently and wait. Be with the students as they start to pack up. Be willing and present for the last minute to answer questions or say hello.

SPIRIT VOYAGER

Call your spirit back into your body.
Silently thank yourself for your courageous work.
This time spent with yourself is never wasted.

BEGIN ANEW

Take one more breath into your body.
Each day we get to wake up and take another breath.
Each day we get to start again.
And mess up again.
Life is in both of these moments.
So when you are ready, let's go out into the world with grateful hearts and open minds.
And begin anew.

THANK YOU

Thank you for showing up today, to carry the torch for this ancient practice.
Thank you for your energy and the willingness to participate with intention and care.
Your contribution to this community that you practice with and to yourself will not go unnoticed.
People are looking to you now, to learn how to live a grace-filled life.
May this practice light your body, mind, and heart and those you are in relationship with today and all days.
(Hare) Om Tat Sat may we awaken to a higher truth
Om: Brahma
Tat: Vishnu
Sat: Shiva
Hare: god

STRONG

This is what the world needs now.
People like you.
Who are willing.
Who are attentive.
Who have courage.
Who are present.

All of these acts contribute not only to your well-being but to all those who you are in relationship with.
Thank you for practicing today.
Your acts reverberate out into the world and contribute to the healing of all.
Namaste the light in me bows to the beautiful noble, light in you.

Nama: bow
As: I
Te: you

A SOUL OF LOVE

I am a soul of love
A heart of peace
A mind of stillness
A being of light
Anonymous

METTA BLESSING

May you be safe
May you be happy
May you be healthy
May you live a life of ease.

ASATOMA

Asatoma: ignorance, not knowing

OM

Asato Maa Sad-Gamaya
Tamaso Maa Jyotir-Gamaya
Mrityor-Maa Amritam Gamaya
Om Shanti, Shanti, Shantihi!

Om
(Let my journey)

Take us from the ignorance to the truth
From darkness to light
And from poison to nectar

SHANTI MANTRA

Shanti: peace
Loka samastha sukhino bhavanthu
Om, shanti, shanti, shanti

May all beings be free
May all beings be happy
May all beings be at peace
Om, peace, peace, peace.

BREATHING POEM

Inhale peace, exhale forgiveness
Inhale acceptance, exhale expectations
Inhale love, exhale hurt
Inhale courage, exhale fear
Inhale
Exhale
Based on the Dalai Lama's Breathing poem

PRAYER OF SAINT FRANCIS

Lord, make me an instrument of your peace
Where there is hatred, let me sow love
Where there is injury, pardon

Where there is doubt, faith
Where there is despair, hope
Where there is darkness, light
And where there is sadness, joy.

GATE GATE
Gate Gate
Parasum gate
Bodhi Svaha!

Gone gone gone
Totally gone to the other side
To join everyone in our community who has walked this path before us
Walk into the light
Oh what a great joy!

From the last mantra of the Heart Sutra

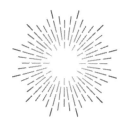

FINAL ODYSSEY

The yoga world is vast and boundless with so much to know and learn. As teachers our tendency can be to keep grasping for more information, knowledge, and experience so one day we can say we have fully arrived and can emblazon the word teacher on our sleeves.

In truth, all of the teachings are information only. We must strive to discern, understand, and integrate the teachings before they can come to life in our classes. Our job is to turn information into rich understanding.

Before I wrote these books, I hosted yoga teachers from around the world in New Zealand. I stood at many airports holding hopeful signs to draw what I so desperately sought closer to me. Each one of them held the 'truth', each one of them put me under a spell. Every time I fell in love. I wanted so desperately to learn and know, to do better.

I collated the information in notebooks; it was a hungry stockpile of words that would eventually become two books.

The thing with falling in love is we think that the person holds what we are looking for, that they complete us. But after ten years of falling in love again and again, I can tell you that it is not that. What I think it is, is that the other person reminds us of what we have forgotten about ourselves. Like a reverse namaste they become bright mirrors that reflect back to us how smart, beautiful, generous, and giving we are. In their presence we are able, capable, present, and loving. When we fall in love, we dust off our shoulders, stand tall, and gleam at all of life. When we are in their presence we are enough. In short, this maturation helps us remember the teachers we were so desperately looking for, we already are.

You embarked on this project when you signed up to be a disciple of yoga. This study is a lifelong, winding, project of seeking that will take many twists and turns towards the truth. As T.S. Eliot tells us—*'We shall not cease from exploration, and the end of all our exploring will be to arrive where we started and know the place for the first time.'*

My wish is that with some extra inspiration you can enmesh something new into what you already do so well. Sometimes all we need is a reminder of what we know and a prompting to teach from that place within that is our inner guide or north star.

May you breathe in inspiration, breath out fear
May each day be another opportunity to fall in love
You have all you need right now—all the knowledge, all the wisdom, all the training.
You hold both the roadmaps and the mazes to your life.
Now it's your turn to pass the batten
From teacher to student to teacher
Your life revolves

BIBLIOGRAPHY

Ashwini, Dhandayutham. "Effect of left & right nostril breathing on R-R interval among adult males – A cross-sectional study." *International Journal of Biomedical Research* 06, no. 2 (February 2015): 87-91. https://ssjournals.com/index.php/ijbr/issue/view/208

Baxter, Bell and Nina Zolotow. *Yoga for Healthy Aging.* Shambala, 2017.

Buddha Dharma Education Association. "The Buddha and His Disciples." Buddhist Studies. 2008. http://www.buddhanet.net/e-learning/buddhism/disciples13.htm

Buettner, Dan. *The Blue Zone Kitchens.* National Geographic, 2019.

Cameron, Julia. *The Artist's Way: A Spiritual Path to Higher Creativity.* Tarcher, 1992.

The Center for Nonviolent Communication (*website*). Updated 2020. https://www.cnvc.org/

Chodron, Pema. *Tonglen: The Path of Transformation.* Vajradhatu Publications, 2001.

Czipin, Jana A. *Ashtanga Yoga: Practice, Theory and Philosophy.* Books on Demand, 2015.

Dale, Cyndi. *The Subtle Body: An Encyclopedia of Your Energetic Anatomy.* Sounds True, 2009.

Damon, Lucy. "Wabi Sabi: The Japanese Philosophy of Embracing Imperfectionism." *Savvy Tokyo*, April 2018. https://savvytokyo.com/wabi-sabi-the-japanese-philosophy-of-embracing-imperfectionism/

Desikachar, T.K.V. *The Heart of Yoga: Developing a Personal Practice.* Inner Traditions International, 1995.

The Yoga Sanctuary. "Exploring the Myths of Asana." Updated 2021. https://www.theyogasanctuary.biz/exploring-the-myths-of-asana-tadasana/

Hanh, Thich Nhat. *Transformation and Healing: Sutra on the Four Establishments of Mindfulness,* 2nd ed. Parallax Press, 2002.

The Hare Krishna Movement. "Lord Krishna Shows the Universal Form Within His Mouth." January 2016, https://theharekrishnamovement.org/2016/01/14/

HARRIS, Gabrielle. *The Language of Yin: Yoga Themes, Sequences, and Inspiration to Bring Your Class to Life & Life to Your Class.* Luminary Press, 2019.

Healing Through Yoga (*website*). https://www.yogacheryl.com/

KABAT-ZINN, Jon. *Wherever You Go There You Are: Mindfulness Meditation in Everyday Life.* Hyperion, 1994.

LEVIN, Stephen M., ed. *Biotensegrity: A New Way of Modeling Biologic Forms.* http://www.biotensegrity.com.

LI, Qing. *Shinrin-Yoku: The Art and Science of Forest Bathing.* Viking, 2018.

———*Forest Bathing: How Trees Can Help You Find Health and Happiness.* Viking, 2018.

Massachusetts Institute of Technology. "MIT Research—Brain Processing of Visual Information." MIT News, 1996. http://news.mit.edu/1996/visualprocessing

MUKUNDANANDA, S. (n.d.). *Bhagavad Gita: Chapter 2, Verse 47.* Retrieved from Bhagavad Gita: https://www.holy-bhagavad-gita.org/chapter/2/verse/47

NEWELL, Zo. "The Mythology Behind Makarasana," *Yoga International,* 2021. https://yogainternational.com/article/view/the-mythology-behind-makarasana-crocodile-pose

PIKÖRN, Isabelle. "Drishti: The Yogic Gaze for Alignment & Awareness." *InsightTimer Blog, 2020.* https://insighttimer.com/blog/drishti-meaning-yoga/

———"The Meaning of Savasana & Why You Should Stay Even Longer." *InsightTimer Blog,* 2020. https://insighttimer.com/blog/savasana-meaning/

*Prana*Shanti Yoga Centre. "Vedantic Philosophy: The Snake and the Rope." 2015. http://pranashanti.com/yoga-stories/vedantic-philosophy-the-snake-and-the-rope/

RATAN, Ravi, and Minoo Ratan. *Journey Through the Chakras.* Rockpool Publishing, 2019.

RICE, Jake. "The Chamsa and the Ahimsa Hand." *Visual Journal of Asian Culture* (blog). January 2015. https://jakericevisualjournal.wordpress.com/2015/01/13/the-chamsa-and-the-ahimsa-hand/

ROCHE, Lorin. *The Radiance Sutras: 12 Gateways to the Yoga of Wonder & Delight.* Sounds True, 2014.

ROSEN, Richard. *Yoga FAQ: Almost Everything You Need to Know About Yoga—from Asanas to Yamas.* Shambala, 2017.

———"Devotion to the Divine," *Yoga Journal,* October 2006, 81.

SARBACKER, Stuart Ray and Kevin Kimple. *The Eight Limbs of Yoga: A Handbook for Living Yoga Philosophy*. North Point Press, 2015.

Satyameva Jayate. (n.d.). Retrieved from Wikipedia: https://en.wikipedia.org/wiki/Satyameva_Jayate

SCHUCMAN, Helen, and William Thetford. *A Course in Miracles*. Foundation for Inner Peace, 2007.

SHAH, Sejal, "The Second Yama of Yoga," *The Art of Living*, June 2018, https://www.artofliving.org/us-en/5-ways-to-practice-satya-being-truthful-second-yama-of-yoga-sutras

STERIOS, Peter, "Do Less with More Awareness: Child's Pose," *Yoga Journal*, August 2007, https://www.yogajournal.com/practice/balasana

STERN, Ken. "Why the Rich Don't Give to Charity," *The Atlantic*, April 2013, https://www.theatlantic.com/magazine/archive/2013/04/why-the-rich-dont-give/309254/

TED. (February 2013). *The Neuroanatomical Transformation of the Teenage Brain | Jill Bolte Taylor* [Video]. YouTube. https://www.youtube.com/watch?v=PzT_SBl31-s

WARE, Bronnie. *The Top Five Regrets of the Dying: A Life Transformed by the Dearly Departing*. California: Hay House Inc., 2012.

Wikipedia, s.v. "Ganga in Hinduism," last modified January 17, 2021, 16:39, https://en.wikipedia.org/wiki/Ganga_in_Hinduism#Crocodile_or_Makra_as_her_vahana

Wisdom Library (*website*). https://www.wisdomlib.org/

INDEX

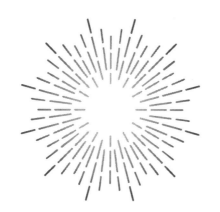

Printed in Great Britain
by Amazon

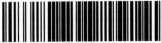

61670948R00221